Eat, Drink and Be Buried

Living Like You Care—The Uncomfortable Reality

By

Manuel Lusquiños

Contents

Dedication i

Acknowledgments ii

About the Author iii

Disclaimer iv

Introduction 1

1 Grim News 5

2 Food Police 6

3 Passive Revolution 8

4 Why Bother? 12

5 Survival 14

6 Who's Running The Show? 16

7 Food Industry 19

8 Nutritionists And Registered Dietitians 22

9 Fitness Trainers 23

10 Science 25

11 Medical Profession 29

12 Pharmaceutical Industry 32

13 Celebrities And Wellness 35

14 Media 38

15 Illusion 46

16 Culture And Tradition 50

17 Excuses 52

18 Standing Alone 65

19 White Flour 68

20 High Fructose Corn Syrup 72

21 Hydrogenated Oil 74

22 Salt 77

23 Sugar 85

24 Artificial Colors 88

25 Chemicals In General 92

26 Weight Loss Obsessed 95

27 Silly Humans 99

28 Buzzwords 106

29 Faulty Reasoning 108

30 Rewiring 114

31 Exercise Is Fun 119

32 Putting It Together 122

33 Exercise In General 131

34 Lifting Weights 136

35 Cardio 145

36 Stretching 153

37 Balance 156

38 No Food Is Perfect 158

39 What To Eat And Drink (Barring Allergies, Other Medical Conditions And Special Needs) 166

40 Defining Good Health... 180
41 Aging... 184
42 Eating And Attitude 196
43 Nutrition 200
44 Accountability 202
45 What To Lose 208
46 Eat At Home 210
47 Diet And Prehistoric Man... 213
48 Trendy Diets And Practices.. 216
49 Idiosyncrasies 219
50 Some Americans 225
51 Fat Pets And Their Humans 227
52 Mindset.. 231
53 Sensitivity Police 241
54 Cost To Healthcare.. 244
55 Childhood Obesity/Overweight... 253
56 In Review 266
Sources... 276

Dedication

To my parents, Luisa and Manuel Lusquiños

Thank you for the push, support and unconditional love. Thank you for repeating the things that really matter. I wish you were both here to see this.

Acknowledgments

Love and a heartfelt thank you to my sister, Maria, for her unwavering encouragement, confidence in me, loyalty and general all-around support.

About the Author

During his law enforcement career, author Manuel Lusquiños was one of the sheep dogs protecting the flock from the wolves. A well-informed flock stands a better chance of survival, not only from the wolves but from itself. This book is the author's attempt to do just that. He was born and raised in Newark, N.J. and currently lives in Pennsylvania.

Disclaimer

The information provided in this book is based solely on the experiences, observations and research of the author. It is only intended to educate, not to recommend treatments or diagnose health threatening conditions, nor is the information herein intended to replace a professional consultation with a medical doctor or other certified healthcare providers. You should consult your physician for all health related matters, including engaging in exercise and dietary changes.

Introduction

The concept of broaching a topic such as living like you care seems painfully axiomatic. After all, doesn't every rational, logical and critically thinking human live this way? Regrettably, no. Therein lies the problem. Based on fifty-plus years of continuing to improve the state of my vitality while observing what the majority is doing, it appears to me that most rational, logical and critically thinking humans, at least when it comes to nutrition, fitness and overall health, have gone the way of the bustle.

Many people say the correct words. Most, undoubtedly, even believe them, but their actions belie their speech. As such, the vast majority stand at a crossroads between a good, healthful life and a sick, miserable existence, which oftentimes leads to an unnecessary and early exit from this mortal plane. Failing to realize this and a reluctance in making health the priority by taking meaningful action, usually leads to a forced realization when it's just too late.

We live in an age of instant and continuous information, with so many people having a pathological relationship with their smartphones, as if the devices were actually an extension of their very bodies. People don't rely on learning, retaining information or innate intelligence anymore because they can simply "Google" anything. Health, nutrition and fitness advice are at our fingertips, in addition to just about all the knowledge that has ever existed about everything, but it seems we are more interested in accessing and viewing cute kitten videos.

Before a problem can be rectified, it must first be recognized. America, and increasingly the rest of the planet, has a dysfunctional relationship with food, fitness and overall health in general. Aside from the unfortunate overweight, underweight and generally unfit individuals whose afflictions are due to medical conditions or poor genetics, how else are we to explain the relentless progress of heart disease, stroke, certain cancers, diabetes, dementia, Alzheimer's disease, osteoporosis, high blood pressure, elevated cholesterol, digestive issues, obesity et cetera? Most of the focus is on the obese. They are growing in number and are easy to spot. But what of the individuals who have medical problems simply because they are overweight, the kind of overweight that is socially accepted, who criticize the obese? What about those thin, unfit and unhealthy folks who believe that thin equals healthy?

It's my belief that eighty percent of what makes us sick and/or kills us is self-induced. These are the behaviors we can change. The other twenty percent are going to eventually do us in, so why worry about what you can't control? Better to deal with the eighty percent by mastering as much of your destiny as possible. Most of the people suffering from various forms of heart disease, diabetes, certain cancers, digestive issues, high blood pressure and so on didn't simply "catch" the illness. Poor choices, stress, substandard food, lack of meaningful exercise, and not enough rest created an environment in their bodies, enabling these afflictions to gain a foothold and flourish. Modern science and medicine have done a pretty good job of controlling and eradicating the pathogens that caused the maladies that we used to "catch." Society and culture have replaced these diseases with the above-mentioned diseases by embracing the standard American diet and attitude. This attitude can be summed up by the old refrain, "Eat, drink and be merry!"

This is a time of hypersensitivity and very thin skin. Most have a fear of criticizing anything or anyone, even when the criticism is well-intentioned. For example, there are some health clubs that boast of being "judgment-free." Sounds like a great idea at first blush until you work out in one of these places. The bowls of Tootsie Rolls on the front counter, the free, white flour bagels with cream cheese and butter offered on every second Tuesday of the month, and the free pizza that can be had on the first Monday of every month are certainly not doing the members any favors. Only then do you see that criticism and judgment are exactly what is needed, with the majority of members having very little idea of proper exercise form, let alone the concept of exercise and nutrition working hand in hand. Most of these unfortunates make no progress even after years of "exercise" and are often at risk for injury. Further, internet postings of grossly obese people, usually scantily clad women, celebrating their individuality are ubiquitous. However, the other side of the story needs to be shouted to the world as well, "Good for you! You're comfortable in your own skin, but chances are high that your health will suffer needlessly due to your corpulence." Inclusivity and acceptance are wonderful concepts, but not at the expense of one's health. People need to know the truth when choosing a path of existence that will probably lead to a negative health outcome. At least the choice will then come after having been exposed to all available facts. Judging one's environment is the result of analyzing information as it's being received. The goal is to make a wise and potentially life-saving decision based on that information.

I judge people who have poor exercise and nutritional habits. For the most part, their overall health is poor and a reflection of these habits. I also judge people with superior exercise and nutritional habits. Not surprisingly, their overall health is usually superior and reflects their habits. Obviously, the more healthful behaviors in which one engages while simultaneously eliminating detrimental behaviors, the greater the odds increase for one to enjoy a long healthful life. There are no guarantees, simply better odds.

Personally, it makes no difference to me how you choose to live your life. As long as what you're doing doesn't affect me, your life choices are none of my business. However, as an observer of the human condition, I have a need to opine on the behaviors of people. Change requires change. In order to improve, you have to look within yourself and ask hard questions, even if you don't like the answers. Do you think it's a good idea to feed your children sugary, salty, artificially colored, fat-laden and chemically infused items masquerading as food? Do you think that allowing your children to drink soda, sports drinks, sweet teas, or energy drinks is a wise choice? Do you think that setting a poor nutrition, fitness and health example for your kids, preparing them for a future complete with the same maladies that afflict you, is what a caring parent does? As far as I'm concerned, the answer to all these questions is an emphatic no! Yet, this is what the majority does.

Most people purchase toxic, pseudo-food from multibillion-dollar corporations, in essence, paying these companies for the right to make them unnecessarily sick and oftentimes contributing to death. These businesses relentlessly plague our media every hour of every day, shamelessly plying their good-for-nothing products. You, being a good American and part of the herd, play right into their hands.

We live in a world in which we control so very little. The idea of controlling your health to the greatest extent possible and perhaps significantly increasing the chances of a satisfactory health outcome should appeal to you. Still, certain people will not be swayed, and that's fine as long as they know the ramifications of their choices. Live and let live. Others think they are on the right path. The "We do meatless Mondays" crowd comes to mind, as do the "I drink only on the weekends" and "I exercise when I have the time" folks. Still, others feel overwhelmed and haven't a clue as to how to begin to change their lives for the better due to the plethora of available information, including good, not-so-good, outright bad, conflicting and seemingly always changing.

The information contained herein is based on years of my own reading, research, training and nutrition experiences, in concert with observing people and listening to their ideas of what constitutes a healthful way of life. I've drawn my own conclusions. The opinions are my own. I've had my fill of endless studies touting the latest and greatest diet, exercise fad or "superfood."

Living a healthful lifestyle should be as mindless as breathing, if you stop listening to all the noise. We're not building a nuclear-powered submarine here. We're simply working on becoming as healthy and fit as we can, given our personal limitations.

This book is for the lost, confused, lazy, overwhelmed, uninformed, delusional, unfit, those who believe they're doing the right thing but aren't, those who know they're not doing the right thing but lie to themselves and those who are willing to buck the societal norms by truly protecting their children from our unfit and unhealthy culture.

Decades ago, when I embarked on this wonderful journey of fitness and health, I had moments of guidance along the way. Today, I continue to learn, reexamine, rethink and change when it is warranted. This book is my way of paying it forward in an effort to provide a general blueprint to improve the health of the common person. It's an attempt to get you to open your eyes and see what you're allowing to be done to you. It's not about gimmicks or quick fixes. It's about desire, commitment, work and will. Once you take responsibility for your own well-being, you begin to take notice of the outside forces that cause you harm. You need to view life from a different perspective. It may cause you some discomfort, but it may also save your life as well as the lives of those you love. I provide this view because I live like I care. I refuse to allow poor food and drink choices, a lack of meaningful exercise and vacuous behaviors and habits to be the cause of my burial. Oh, I'll be buried alright, but I won't be digging my own grave.

1

Grim News

Let's get the bad news out of the way first. No matter who you are or how you live, healthfully, unhealthfully or somewhere in between, we all have an expiration date. Yes, sadly, we all die. We can't do anything about the dying part, but we have a great deal of control over the living part. I find it astonishing that the majority take what was once a viable, vibrant living organism with so much hope and promise for the future and transform it into a sickly, medicated, unfit, self-destructive meat puppet.

I'm well aware some individuals prefer hotdogs, ice cream, deli meats, salt, sugar, soda, cheesy pizza, fatty snacks, animal products, alcohol, coffee and tobacco to healthful fare such as vegetables, fruits, whole grains, legumes, nuts and seeds. That is their prerogative. People should live as they wish.

Some have expressed they would rather live a shorter life while eating as much of whatever they desire, whenever they desire. However, my encounters with people have led me to believe that the individuals preferring substandard food, while realizing the dire health implications of ingesting such food, are in the minority. Most people want it both ways. They want to be fit, healthy, attractive and confident but are unwilling to put in the effort required. Worse are those who delude themselves into believing they are doing all the right things to reach their health and fitness goals yet remain perplexed and frustrated when the goals are never attained.

The choice is yours. You can take as much control of your health and fitness outcome as possible, or you can leave it to chance by engaging in habits that will most likely lead to unnecessary illness, pain, premature aging and early death.

2
Food Police

Let me be clear: I'm not the food police. Eat as you wish. I'm an opinionated observer and commentator. However, changes need to be made in order to transform our unhealthful culture into a healthful one. As such, it is my opinion that parents making poor food choices for their children are doing those children a grave disservice by setting the kids up for a future of easily avoidable diseases. Further, school cafeteria food is, for the most part, abysmal. As if this were not bad enough, vending machines dispensing soda and cheap junk foods have no place in educational institutions, nor do classroom junk food parties. It is the job of schools to encourage and inspire learning and enlightenment for the betterment of the individual as well as the whole of society— tomorrow's leaders. The phrase "tomorrow's leaders" is often quoted but rendered meaningless if schools do nothing but continue to indoctrinate students into the accepted and approved behaviors of a sick society.

Hospitals and senior care facilities are two more places where it seems painfully obvious that health-promoting sustenance would be the order of the day. If you've ever visited such an institution and have even a rudimentary understanding of proper nutrition, you are clearly aware that this is not the case. Sadly, this is true despite the fact that both usually have a registered dietician on staff.

I have no enthusiasm for the government to ban what I consider to be unacceptable foods from supermarkets. Far too many unintended consequences usually arise when the government steps in to "fix" a problem. I don't believe in a nanny state. What I would enjoy is seeing companies change their practices due to people avoiding the injurious products these businesses produce. Admittedly, I would not shed a tear and would, in fact, be elated to see certain products and companies go away, dying a natural death due to a lack of interest by savvy consumers.

We need to change the food and fitness culture, but we don't need food police. Instead, what the government should provide is an honest, urgent and unwavering campaign to increase public awareness through education, making health through proper nutrition and fitness a priority instead of a niche topic.

Understandably, standardized food nutrition labels should be required on all packaged foods. There should be restrictions on marketing junk food to children. Nutrition and fitness education classes should be required in public schools, K-12. Medical schools need to wake up and provide our future doctors with a robust block of instruction on nutrition and exercise and how they relate to disease. Healthcare providers, in general, need to be much better informed about nutrition and exercise. They need to understand and promote disease prevention. Only then will we genuinely possess a healthcare system, rather than the illness management structure that currently afflicts us.

3

Passive Revolution

Supply and demand is a basic economic principle. If there's a big enough demand for a product, you'll find someone more than happy to sell it to you. Most of the edible and drinkable products available in the majority of supermarkets we are familiar with, including those supermarkets with a reputation for wholesome fare, are inferior foods. There are more aisles of highly processed, salt, sugar, artificial sweetener, fat and chemically infused pseudo-foods for sale than health-promoting foods. Throw in all the foods derived from animals, and it's no wonder why we are so unhealthy.

Have you ever strolled down the cereal aisle in one of these places? It's not much different than walking into a candy store. They could do away with 99% of the products on display here. The marketing behind these cereals, and I'm using the word cereals very loosely here, is stunningly brilliant. What little kid would not be drawn to the bright and colorful packaging depicting familiar cartoon characters? Their parents also fall prey to sharp marketing ploys, but in their case, they manifest in the form of exaggerated health claims on adult-appropriate packaged items. The boxes shout out the presence of fiber, protein, bran, flax seeds and so on. They claim to be heart-healthy, natural and organic. The reality is that cereals marketed to children are mostly sugar, artificial colors, difficult-to-pronounce chemicals and sometimes actually contain marshmallows. The cereals marketed to adults may be a little better, but a little better does not qualify as healthful. Add to the equation that most boxed cereals are preserved with BHT (Butylated hydroxytoluene), and healthful is not the first adjective that comes to mind.

Admittedly, some of these products may contain some vitamins, minerals and other nutrients, but the minuscule benefits are overwhelmingly outweighed by the negatives. The best cereals on the market generally contain one ingredient, a whole grain and sometimes a few whole grains in combination. Often, healthful, whole-grain cereals are combined with seeds like chia or hemp. These are also good choices. Look for cereals like whole wheat, whole oats, whole quinoa, whole millet, whole amaranth, whole kamut and whole buckwheat, to name a few. Added salt, sugar, artificial sweeteners, oils, colorings, chemical preservatives, or other science lab ingredients may make the product more attractive to children and childlike adults, but the objective here is health.

The soda aisle is another area that's a waste of space from a health standpoint, though certainly not from a business angle. Soda, diet or otherwise, is water infused with sugar or artificial sweeteners and chemicals that do not even serve to quench your thirst. When you ingest soda, you are drinking useless, harmful liquid calories and chemicals that have no nutritional value. Make your fuel count. Drinking water is the best liquid fuel choice. As far as solid fuels go, derive them from healthful, nutritious sources such as plant-based products—fruits, vegetables, whole grains, raw and/or dry roasted nuts and seeds, beans and legumes. Food and liquids are the power sources that make you run. You may be made of flesh, but you are a meat machine. Utilizing the best propellants available increases your chances of running more efficiently, longer and with fewer breakdowns. This results in fewer visits to the shop or, in the case of humans, the doctor. Follow this advice, and you'll improve your odds of remaining in the game of life and avoiding the scrap heap until it's truly your time.

In addition to the cereal and soda aisles, the snack aisle is another death trap. Cheery-looking packages of chips, pretzels and other crunchy things oozing chemicals, salt, sugar and artery-clogging fat beckon from their perches. The purveyors of these toxic concoctions oftentimes scam gullible consumers by presenting labels announcing healthful sounding claims such as, "Low Sodium," "Low Calorie," "No Salt," "Baked Not Fried," "Whole Grain" and other supposedly healthful proclamations. Don't be fooled. Remember, the goal of these companies is to separate you from your hard-earned dollars, not to enhance your health and well-being. All of these products contain a combination of, or at least one of these ingredients: chemicals, salt, sugar, artificial sweeteners, artificial coloring agents, oil and other fats. Even if they've added only one of the aforementioned ingredients to a whole grain or other wholesome product, they've ruined the wholesomeness of that product. You can easily see an example of nutritious food being destroyed when attempting to purchase a jar of unadulterated raw or dry roasted nuts or seeds. These are very difficult to find, and when you do find them, their presence is overwhelmed by the ubiquity of nuts and seeds that have been rendered into junk food status due to the addition of, at the very least, salt. When considering the oils, sweeteners and such, you'd do well to pass by these products in the snack aisle.

The cookie, cake, candy and bread aisles share a commonality with the cereal and snack food aisle. Generally, all of them are simply a combination of sickening ingredients, which are sometimes added to a well-recognized nutritious ingredient—think salt, sugar and artificial dye added to a whole-grain product. Read the labels.

Other inferior food-like products that can be found in almost all supermarkets include salad dressings, canned vegetables, canned fruits, microwavable ready-made meals and usually any product that has been mixed, combined or prepared in any way for your convenience. Even if the product boasts organic or all-natural packaging, pay no mind. Again, read the ingredients on the label. What's the point if an organic product is still laden with salt, sugar, fat and chemicals? Further, don't be fooled by the marketing ploys of purveyors of health food products such as protein bars, protein powders and other healthful sounding fare. Most of these items should be in the candy aisle. Remember, the best products don't contain added salt, sugar, oil or chemicals. Again, calling something vegan or labeling it organic or all-natural is meaningless if it contains these additives.

Power, position, authority, whatever name it goes by, does not readily give up its status. The mighty food industry, along with its lobbyists and other allies, depends on the ignorance and laziness of the citizenry. They know what makes people tick. Most people demand and receive lousy food because the priorities of the majority are convenience, speed and the path of least resistance. The issue of health and fitness is an abstract notion that doesn't really gain any traction until health and fitness are lost. Those in charge give the masses just what they ask for and tell them exactly what they want to hear. This assures that those at the top will remain there. Our leaders don't have the political will or incentive to change our disease-promoting food culture because not enough people demand that they do so. The notion of the government being there to serve the general welfare of the population and the idea that all food producers have our best interests in mind when they promote their products are no more than warm and fuzzy ideals. From a health perspective, the reality is something else entirely.

With all the issues that people get worked up about enough to organize, protest, march, write letters to editors and congressmen and generally create an uproar, where is the moral outrage and incredulity when it comes to the state of our food and fitness? While it's a noble pursuit to save the world from the ravages of climate change, preserve endangered species, clean polluted air and water, ensure equality among the races and sexes, prevent thermonuclear annihilation, show compassion to immigrants and the homeless, ensure fair wages, reduce the gap between the haves and the have nots, promote democracy or whichever cause gets your blood boiling enough to do something about it, what's the point if you're only going to destroy yourself anyway? The first thing that needs saving is you. Then, you can move on to your issue of choice.

As wonderful as it would be to witness an overt revolution against a culture that encourages the consumption of foods that contribute to diseases, think marches, letters to politicians and policymakers, protests, editorial letter write-in campaigns to major newspapers, social media blitzes, well, I'm sure you get the idea, none of it is necessary in order to help yourself. You can protest just as well and in a less labor-intensive fashion by doing so passively and very quietly. Simply, don't buy bad food. Don't waste your money on food that is harming you. Don't pay the producers of lousy food for the privilege of killing you. It's senseless. And the remark that I so often hear about how expensive it is to eat healthfully is a myth. Healthful food is no more or less expensive than inferior food. It just depends on what you buy. You can make a very healthful meal from a variety of whole grains, beans and vegetables. These are not expensive items. Time and time again, as I wait at the checkout at the grocery store, I observe what the people ahead of me are buying. Usually, it's mostly inferior food permeated with a pestilential brew of the additives I warned you to be wary of earlier. To add insult to injury, the shoppers I've observed, usually pay more for their food than do I for mine. Protest loudly and obviously or passively and quietly. If you stop purchasing bad food, slowly but surely, not unlike cigarettes, bad food will, if not entirely disappear, be relegated to a lower status. Demand healthful food, and you'll get it. You can be part of the problem or the solution. The choice is yours.

4

Why Bother?

I'm not religious, but if religion and blind faith work for you, so be it. If you're an atheist and that gives you peace, embrace it. If more people were honest with themselves, they'd probably fall into my category, that of hopeful agnostic. None of us know of the existence of God or what happens, if anything, other than decomposition after death, but the idea of an eternal afterlife, I must admit, has its appeal. This is especially true if you consider the fact that no matter how you lead your life, only a small percentage of humans manage to live to 100 years and beyond, with the outer limits of human existence at this time being about 120 years. Philosophically speaking and bearing in mind that all things are relative, even living to 120 years is a blink in the grand scale of the universe.

Perhaps that's why I'm less dogmatic than I used to be about health and fitness. As I stated earlier, what you do with your life is your business. But, your decisions are better, based on reliable information and reality, not trends, marketing or what everyone else is doing. The most important thing is to give children a fair chance to make choices as they grow older by educating them honestly while they are young, keeping their best interests in mind. As adults, if they make choices that go counter to living a fit and healthful life, yet these decisions bring them pleasure, who is anyone to tell them to do otherwise? We're not here that long, so be content.

Humans have puffed themselves up into a state of hyper-importance. Yes, we are the lords of the earth, although every now and again, a much less bombastic, pathogenic creature comes along to knock us down a peg. Regardless, as far as we're concerned, we're at the top of the food chain. No need to mention all the advances in science, technology and medicine that humans have made throughout history, for they are well documented. Yet, I can't help but go back to that 100-120 years of maximum life expectancy. We work, scrape, suffer, cry, worry, laugh, love and die. What's the point? Why are we here? Perhaps nothing really matters. I mean, 100-120 years? Big deal. Ninety-nine percent of humanity is forgotten as the decades go by. When all the people who knew you while you were alive come to their end, it's as if you never existed. That makes us sound much less important, in my view. As such, why bother being concerned with exercise and good nutrition, right? It depends on what your priorities are and what you value most. Do you prefer the pleasure of eating and drinking as much as you want, of anything you want, thus dramatically

12

increasing your odds of contracting preventable diseases, accelerating your cellular aging and courting premature death? Do you prefer doing everything within your power to always be in your best physical condition? Are you a disciple of moderation? Only you can answer where you fit in on the health and fitness continuum.

Unfortunately, most people delude themselves. They want it both ways. That much bandied-about word, moderation, mentioned above, comes to mind. It simply doesn't work. Moderation is generally the last vestige of weak, excuse-making justifiers. These are people who don't have the strength of their convictions. If you want to achieve your best personal health and fitness, you don't go about it in a moderate fashion. This idea is analogous to driving moderately. A person driving and observing the rules of the road moderately well is more likely to be involved in an accident than a person doing all he can to be a safe driver. Those individuals who drive carelessly and recklessly are similar to people who eat carelessly and recklessly. The odds are less in their favor for a successful health outcome. Of course, you can be the most prudent driver on the road, and this does not prevent a bad driver from hitting you head-on. Things happen. Nevertheless, I remain a strong advocate of keeping the odds in my favor. It's the best you can do because nothing is perfect. You would do well to do the same if you view your health and well-being as a precious gift to be preserved.

You should bother being as healthy and fit as possible. Why? For the brief time that we are on Earth, no reasonable person wants to suffer. Exercise and proper eating help maintain a healthy you. Life is hard enough. Should we make it harder by aiding and abetting the various forces beyond our control that cause us harm? Heart disease, various cancers, diabetes, stroke, high blood pressure and arteriosclerotic diseases are, more often than not, caused by poor food choices and a paucity of meaningful exercise. As such, they are often preventable. By and large, we arrive at our present condition based on the choices we've made. I'm certain that most relatively intelligent, logical people, if given a choice between rotting away in a medical facility, connected to various pieces of life-sustaining machinery, for the last 10 years of life or living to a healthy, fit, 120 years, independent, lucid, full of vitality and feeling great one minute then suddenly dropping dead the next, would opt for the latter. Think it through. Minimize the suffering.

5

Survival

If we eliminate reality television, Monday Night Football, The View, thumbing our cellphones, hanging on every word and action of celebrities and the nightly glass of Merlot, what are each one of us, as living biological organisms, really trying to do? Survive. It's as simple as that. The rest is mostly useless noise. Unfortunately, because so many people are incapable of dealing with the realities of life, the mostly useless noise is akin to the song of the Sirens, which, figuratively speaking, causes us to crash into the rocks.

Our will to survive has been supplanted by an irrepressible desire for instant gratification. Human beings are inherently lazy. We want it fast, easy, convenient and cheap. Too often, we don't think before we act because we're on autopilot. Our limited attention spans are taken advantage of by advertisers. For example, have you ever noticed that as you are comfortably settled on your couch, not five minutes into the most tediously hyped ballgame of the season, the announcer begins to excitedly promote next week's game? We are constantly encouraged, cajoled, pressured and pushed into the next best game, event, holiday, season, automobile, activity or behavior, even as we are in the midst of the latest thing to which we mindlessly succumbed at the behest of all the blathering marketers. All this while we are simultaneously being told to live in the moment, to be present.

The ebbing in our collective will to continue existing has been incentivized, aided and abetted by a cultural attitude that emphasizes buying things we don't really need, consuming food and drink which, at the least, contribute to preventable diseases and, at the worst, contribute to death. Further, we are coaxed into engaging in activities that can only be characterized as being from mindless to dangerous. To what end? On the one hand, the businesses pushing all this nonsense are successful in getting you to purchase their products, while on the other hand, you become distracted from the one thing most people have a hard time coming to terms with—their own mortality. So everybody's happy, right? As far as the businesses go, they'll remain happy as long as you keep giving them your money. You'll only remain happy until, most likely, the inevitable medical event occurs as a result of the foolish choices you've made. You thought what you were doing was living and enjoying, not so much when you get a less than favorable medical diagnosis that was entirely preventable.

Once bodily systems begin to break down and fail, we are suddenly faced with the looming possibility that we may not be long for this world. Sometimes, we are given a temporary reprieve, and a handful of us embrace the opportunity and turn our lives toward health and survival. Regrettably, most return to business as usual. This latter group, yet again, allows itself to be manipulated and encouraged through propaganda and subliminal advertising into paying, in one form or another, the entities that benefit from their self-inflicted maladies.

You can't begin to live and enjoy until you first learn to survive. After you learn to survive, then comes the living. If you work hard and have a bit of luck, you will then thrive. Unfortunately, most humans are like the grasshopper in Aesop's fable. The grasshopper spent the summer singing and having fun, while the ant spent his summer gathering and storing food in preparation for winter. When the bitter winter arrived, the ant was in good shape while the grasshopper was dying from starvation and begged the ant for food. People are commonly poor at preparation and maintenance. Think about all the people who wait until their child is in high school before they start saving for that child's college education. The same goes for those who are on the cusp of retirement before it dawns on them that they had better start saving money for that long anticipated and what should be a carefree time of life. They habitually respond more robustly to drama, catastrophe and spectacle by hand wringing, worry and panic even though by that point, it's usually too late. It's no different than waiting until you're sick to realize that your health matters. Prepare; don't panic.

There are many enablers in our culture masquerading as supporters, which inhibit our survival. These include but are not limited to food producers, food sellers, advertisers, the media, the pharmaceutical-medical industry and the government. This does not serve as an excuse to those who see themselves as victims of a master conspiracy by these establishments to derail their health and continuance. Rather, it is a sobering commentary that our best chance for survival ultimately rests on our own shoulders. Self-reliance and taking responsibility are the keys.

6

Who's Running The Show?

An erroneous thought process routinely undertaken by the average citizen is that he's in charge of his own life. No one wants to play the part of the mark, the patsy. Yet, millions do so every day. As an example, with the abundance of information available on all media outlets advising us on how not to be scammed, cheated, lied to and manipulated, so many of us continue to make choices detrimental to our health and welfare by freely giving out personal information to con artists. We readily and unquestioningly follow the advice of doctors, lawyers, clergy, celebrities and anyone else we perceive to be infallible and to have our best interests in mind. All this blind faith occurs without the least bit of critical thought on our part. Combining this blind faith with people who are uncomfortable with plain speaking, questioning the status quo, worrying about what others will think of them and typically being afraid to stand alone creates the perfectly malleable consumer.

I have nothing personal against doctors, lawyers, clergy or celebrities. The problem is we tend to believe people because of their titles or status, not because of their credibility. However, these individuals are human and suffer the same foibles as the rest of us. My point is that we are too quick to believe and to want to believe, especially if the belief brings us satisfaction.

It can be reasonably stated that the wellness industry includes components of, but is not limited to, marketing the businesses of nutrition, fitness, medicine and pharmacology, and as such, is a multibillion-dollar per year behemoth. It is an industry rife with snake oil salesmen. It's a pleasant, albeit naive, thought to believe that these bodies collectively exist solely to serve our overall health interests. Mostly, the wellness industry, as with all businesses, is motivated by making money. A lot of money. Lobbyists, marketers and advertisers are the foot soldiers waging the battle to get hold of your dollars. And they are winning. How else is one to explain the sales of what some of you may be too young to remember, the Pet Rock, the Invisible Dog Leash, the 1960s "Fat Burning"/Shaker Machine or the vibrating "Slimming" Belt, guaranteed to tone those abs and reduce your waist? In the 1950s, some doctors were paid shills for cigarette companies in an attempt to convince the impressionable public of the benefits of smoking. Advertisements are made to be very compelling in an effort to get us to behave or not behave in a certain manner. From print to online and everything in between, the pitchmen set the trap, lure us in and wait for us to take the bait. They prey on our emotions by utilizing music, color and fun. Advertisers do extensive studies and market analyses on what motivates us. They're extremely skilled at predicting what we will do before we do it. The aphorism that "There is a sucker born every minute" has been attributed to P.T. Barnum and a handful of other men throughout history. Whoever was responsible for uttering that phrase was being conservative.

Generally, the combination of a multibillion-dollar per year business, in this case the wellness industry, in league with the power of government, usually results in an unsatisfactory outcome for the common citizenry. Most people would probably say that the job of the government is to protect its citizens and provide for their general welfare. This is done by creating and implementing policy intended to serve the interests of the majority. I contend that the main job of government is to remain in existence. Therefore, the most important job performed by a politician is that of campaigning to be reelected if he is the incumbent or to be elected if he does not currently hold office. Routinely, politicians will say just about anything necessary to be elected, reelected or remain in office. Political party affiliation makes no difference because whether Democrat or Republican, each is but a different side of the same coin, with the minor parties being the coin's edge. Politics is like any other white-collar career and mostly a good job if you can get it. The pensions and perks are exceedingly attractive, especially at the upper strata of governmental service.

Politicians and anyone else you perceive to be a member of an elevated caste are simply humans like us. Some may be better known and have greater wealth, but they are plagued by the same shortcomings. These officials need to be held to a higher standard of behavior than the masses due to the gravitas of their respective positions—that of serving the safety and health of their constituency. It is routine to see many of our elected officials fall far short of any idealized higher standard in general terms. Therefore, it's no surprise to see their tepid efforts, assuming that they are even making attempts to repair our mostly overweight, out-of-shape and overmedicated society.

Far too many citizens take our leaders at face value. "They wouldn't say that if it weren't true" is a phrase that, astonishingly, is expressed by so many of the guileless. This, despite the well known facts that our government permitted slavery, didn't allow women to vote, imprisoned thousands of Japanese American citizens during World War II simply because they were Japanese, was responsible for racial segregation, advised school children during the Cold War that they would be safe hiding under their desks in the event of a thermonuclear attack, told us that the war in Vietnam was a police action necessary to stifle the proliferation of communism via the domino theory, conducted the Tuskegee Syphilis Study whereby hundreds of African-American men with the disease were left untreated for the benefit of scientific study, advised us that the air at Ground Zero was safe to breath after 9/11, told us that Iraq was invaded because they were in possession of weapons of mass destruction, allowed corporate water and air pollution to continue unchecked for years, put a man on the moon over 50 years ago and has had a manned space station orbiting above us since 2000 but wants us to believe that getting 30 miles per gallon of gasoline in our family vehicles is cause for celebration because no technology could possibly exist that would give us triple-digit miles per gallon of gas. Call me cynical, but I think there might be something going on between big oil companies and the government. The equation is simple: government + big business = power & money.

Big business contributes money to political campaigns in order to curry favor with elected officials. Politicians don't have the will to inhibit the profits of the very companies that helped get them elected in the first place and might potentially help again in the future. It's not politically expedient to double-cross your allies. In addition, big business predicts our every move and mesmerizes us with hype about whatever it is they wish us to purchase while cleverly manipulating us into believing the purchase decision is entirely our own. This, compounded by the government telling us what it thinks we want to hear and what it believes we are entitled to hear, does not set the stage for a transparent and honest discussion on how best to revamp our disease-promoting cultural norms. One need only look at the various permutations of the federal government's food pyramid and plate. The revisions that have taken place over time to these so-called nutritional guidelines were not done solely out of a concern for public health. The bigger concern was to avoid antagonizing the meat and dairy industries. As a whole, the government and big business don't care about us as individuals and that's fine by me because I'm not naive enough to expect them to. We are no more than a means to their respective ends. Once we embrace this idea, we can move on and begin to take responsibility for our own well-being. At that point, if the government or business offers us something that truly benefits our existence, we can utilize that something. Effectively, they become a means to our collective ends. Look at it as a leveling of the playing field. Force the government and businesses to serve us by not accepting inferior products or policies from either of them. Take charge and run your own show. Your life depends on it.

7

Food Industry

When I say the food industry, I'm referring to food markets, restaurants (both fast food and upscale), farmers, packagers and the rest of the interconnected web of businesses that produce, package, deliver and sell what we eat. Their sole purpose is to make a profit. Most of them are beholden to stockholders, the pressures of Wall Street and managing the bottom line. If given a choice between profiting handsomely by producing a salty, fatty, sugary food product that no one in his right mind would remotely consider a benefit to the health of humanity or profiting somewhat by offering a healthful food product, the salty, fatty and sugary food will always win out. It's just good business.

The key here for the food industry is how to lure the consumer into purchasing inferior food. In this instance, my use of the term inferior food refers mostly to heavily processed, prepackaged items, many of which I mentioned previously. These include standard as well as vegetarian and vegan selections. They encompass but are not limited to cereals, soups, chips, breads, bakery products, salad dressings, sodas, luncheon meats, nut butters, jellies, sauces, spreads, dips, grains, vegetables, fruits and many more items.

This is where advertising plays a role. Advertisers know that different things motivate different people. When it comes to food, most people operate with their reptilian brains—I'm hungry, the food is there, it looks good, it smells good, it tastes good, I'm stuffed—very basic. These individuals are a food producer and advertiser's dream because they're easy to capture with simple bait. Any combination of fat, salt and sugar added to just about anything within reason that a generic human can fit into his mouth will do. Some individuals prove to be more elusive prey. However, by the time a few artificial colors and chemicals providing enticing aromas and a nice mouth feel are added, compounded by suitable, attention-grabbing packaging and a catchy jingle, even these somewhat more elusive prey are no match for the relentless advertisers.

But what of bigger game? What is the food industry and its advertisers to do with that scant and ever so slowly growing number of the population, who are beginning to show an interest and concern about what they eat? For this most elusive quarry the best bait has proven to be health claims on packages. The providers of what we eat are always on the watch for new trends, healthful or not, just profitable. Words like healthy, organic, natural, sustainable, free-range, locally sourced, fair trade, wellness and earth friendly, to name but a handful, have been bleeding into the daily lexicon for quite a few years. For the most part, those who embrace these types of terms are still considered extremists. They are looked upon as liberal, fringe members of the general population who most likely listen to NPR.

Shrewd food makers and marketers, however, see opportunities to add to their already overflowing coffers. When next you visit the food market, take a good look at the health and earth-friendly claims popping up on the packaging of so many items now available. This isn't simply happenstance. The industry is well aware that there is money to be made in the business of wellness which includes both humanity and the environment. Foods with labels proclaiming heart healthy, low sodium, cholesterol-free, more fiber, added vitamins, fat-free, sugar-free and more vie for the attention of the health conscious. I've seen "no cholesterol" labels on fresh vegetables and fruits. These are foods that never have contained, nor will they ever contain cholesterol. I would be the first to suggest you consume plenty of fresh produce because it's an excellent food source. But to affix a "no cholesterol" label on fresh fruits and vegetables should be an insult to your intelligence. Cholesterol is found only in animals, not plants. This is pretty basic.

The gluten-free foods and, in many cases, entire sections devoted solely to these foods, which have sprouted up like weeds in so many supermarkets, are bemusing. "Gluten Free" has become still another trendy buzzword hooking the dupable among us. Gluten is nothing more than a combination of proteins found in the endosperm of various cereal grains. This grouping of proteins is what gives dough its stretch and supplies most of the protein in wheat. People who are sensitive or allergic to gluten and especially those suffering from celiac disease, in which case an individual can become seriously ill, need to avoid gluten-containing foods and drinks. It's no different than a person having a severe allergy to peanuts or having a seriously unhealthy reaction to other foods, which can sicken and potentially kill a person coping with food-induced maladies.

Simply put, if the food in question and your biological makeup are incompatible, causing you to develop a medical condition and even threatening your life, prudence would dictate that you avoid that food at all costs. However, if the food causes you no problem, then there is no problem. Advertisers give that supposedly health-aware demographic the sense that gluten is synonymous with poison. It's no more or less a poison than a peanut. Not surprisingly, the food industry and its public relations machine will mine its dollars from whichever demographic is willing to turn them over.

Fast food restaurants, not wanting to miss out on their own opportunity to cash in, have also jumped on the health bandwagon. In addition to their usual selection of disease-promoting fare, many now offer what they are touting as more healthful options, such as meatless or plant-based burgers. To reiterate, it's not because they're concerned about public health. Nor is public health a concern of restaurants serving bar food or upscale cuisine, even though more healthful selections are becoming increasingly prevalent in most food serving establishments. They all want a piece of your wallet and are willing and able to cast a wide net in order to ensnare as many consumers as possible, no matter what they eat. Eaters beware.

Functional foods, also referred to as nutraceutical foods, are another chic designation applied to a variety of foods that have potential health benefits beyond simple nutrition. For example, leafy green vegetables such as kale, spinach and chard are viewed as functional foods because they provide calcium for good bone health, in addition to a variety of vitamins and other minerals essential for our bodies to perform optimally. Oats are also considered a functional food for their known ability to help lower cholesterol. Generally speaking, vegetables, fruits, nuts, seeds, legumes and whole grains all fall under the functional foods umbrella. I encourage all who are mindful of their well-being to eat more of these health-promoting foods.

The problem with functional foods is when the food industry steps in and designates a food product a functional food, which has no business being labeled as such. Think about it. How many low-quality food products have you come across that used to stand alone in all their uselessness? Suddenly, they've been recast as "health foods" by incorporating beneficial ingredients such as fiber, calcium, flax seeds, whole wheat, vitamins and a variety of others. They can be easily found at your local grocery store. Infusing an inherently inferior food with a healthful ingredient doesn't transform the inferior food into something acceptable. Bad food should never be the delivery vehicle for life-enhancing ingredients. Care about and respect your body by demanding and eating only good food. In a worst-case scenario, eat only the best food available. Don't settle for less.

8

Nutritionists And Registered Dietitians

Professional nutritionists and registered dietitians have forgotten more about the chemical components of foods than I will ever know. How they interact with each other and within the human body remains a mystery to me. These people are well-educated and highly knowledgeable in their field. Many have practices where they see clients or patients. Some are consultants, authors and college professors with PhDs, or they work for large institutions and companies in need of the services of a nutrition expert. These include: schools, hospitals, nursing homes, airlines, public health clinics, government agencies, NPOs (nonprofit organizations), prisons, cafeterias, etc.

I've experienced hospital food as a patient, and I've seen it served while visiting patients. I know what type of food is being served in public schools. I've seen various menus from long-term care facilities. I've been exposed to airline food on numerous occasions. Another thought is the quality of food served in prisons. If so much of the food served to our most vulnerable population in schools, nursing homes and hospitals is inferior, how healthful can prison food be? Prisoners don't have a prayer. This is another good reason not to get arrested. Even with nutrition experts on staff, a good portion of the food at these institutions is deplorable.

Something is obviously, at least to me, very wrong here. Registered Dietitians working for large institutions want to keep their jobs just like everyone else. I've spoken to some who have been quite honest in admitting that they simply spout the party line but don't actually believe what their superiors instruct them to say. I've been to presentations of other nutrition authorities who were overweight, terribly out of shape and espoused the mantra of moderation. In short, having a nutrition expert on staff or consulting doesn't guarantee a nutritious food result.

9

Fitness Trainers

As a result of our common mortal flaws, fitness trainers, as with everyone else, are not created equally. I know a few very competent trainers who have the strength of their convictions, do not suffer fools and care deeply about helping their clients become the best version of themselves. Good trainers teach clients how to navigate the gym environment. Also, they incorporate nutrition lessons and more during their client's training sessions because they know that exercise, nutrition and nuanced gym comportment work together to produce the best possible results. If you're in the market for a trainer, this is the type of person you want to hire.

On the other hand, many trainers, who, for the most part, know more about exercise, nutrition and fitness than the average person, don't always put their knowledge to its best use. Even after receiving an instructor's certification, many retain false notions about exercise and food. I've seen poor demonstrations of exercise techniques in gyms throughout the country by trainers who are being paid by their clients to know better. Much of the dietary advice I've overheard being dispensed to unsuspecting and desperately unfit customers by their instructors is disheartening. I've witnessed some trainers engage their clients in jovial conversations while the clients were doing all they could just to eke out the prescribed number of repetitions on a piece of gym equipment, with free weights and on floor exercise. Many trainers and clients sit around for extended periods of time, occupying equipment that others are waiting to use. This time spent talking, laughing and basically engaging in inane banter is far more time than is necessary for the client to recover from the previous set of exercise.

So many trainers, being clueless themselves, fail to educate their customers on proper gym etiquette. This includes habits such as stripping weights from barbells and machines when you finish with them, as well as returning weight plates, dumbbells and other gym gear to their properly designated racks or spots. Teaching people to wipe off sweaty equipment, to refrain from crossing between you and a mirror you're standing close to while observing your form in the midst of a set, alerting clients to the inconsiderate behavior of leaving their personal workout paraphernalia spread out on multiple pieces of equipment, dissuading trainees from carrying on loud cell phone conversations as well as human to human conversations while in close proximity to people who are actually focussed on training and many other tips on the way one should conduct oneself in a public space, specifically, a gym in this instance, are concepts and behaviors that are often beyond the grasp of trainers.

Even though these modes of conduct are common sense, they need to be reinforced because many people appear to exhibit a lack of just that, common sense. Not educating clients properly sets the stage for wave after wave of uninformed, disruptive and irritating gym members to clash with those members who are in the know. Avoid clueless trainers and clueless clients for a better workout and a more satisfying gym experience.

10

Science

In a perfect world, the job of science would be to seek truth and knowledge without the encumbrances of prejudice, emotion, greed and other pressures from outside forces. Unfortunately, perfection is not one of the characteristics of our world, scientists included. Like every other human being, they also suffer from the same weaknesses and flaws, make mistakes and at times, show poor judgment. Many in the scientific community depend on grants to conduct and continue their research. When it's reported that a particular scientific study is touting the incredible health benefits of one food or another, the first thing we need to ask is, "Who sponsored the study?" It's important to know who's paying the scientist, what he gains by supporting or vilifying the food being studied and if he has other agendas.

Sometimes, scientists have less than noble reasons for their conclusions, but other times, they simply get it wrong. People are going to believe what they want to believe to be true, as goes the saying. No matter how questionable and, at times, outlandish the determination of a study may be, if it fits within an individual's framework, it becomes gospel. This is especially true in the nutrition/fitness field, where the majority of the unfit are always looking for that elusive magic bullet. Few people are more desperately gullible than the unfit who are overweight, searching for the magic cure for their condition. Many are convinced by research studies that the cure requires no more than simply swallowing a pill or drinking a liquid and going to bed. These individuals hope that these remedies will result in a miraculous weight loss, freeing them from further responsibility. They happily believe their problem is solved.

Remember many years ago when science told us that popping salt pills during sweaty athletic practices was a good thing? Do you recall the news reports from a few decades ago that high doses of niacin were a miracle cholesterol-lowering strategy? These two fell out of favor. Consuming extra beta-carotene, red wine, coffee, chocolate, soy, vitamins, organic foods, red meat and animal products in general are just a smattering of the overwhelming, inexhaustible amount of nutritionally controversial topics of research and study that rain down upon us in torrents, seemingly every day. What was good for us yesterday is bad for us today. What was traditionally considered bad for us yesterday is good for us today.

A study is only as good as the scientist behind it. I believe that most scientists are well-intentioned and perform superior work. I harbor this belief while being ever vigilant for study sponsors. I don't put too much credence in the meat industry or the dairy industry, for example, to pay for studies concerning the wisdom of consuming their respective products. It's quite obvious that if you're the one controlling the study, you're not going to shoot yourself in the foot. Science can justify anything. It's all about how the information is presented. If there exists a study praising a specific nutrient or food, there undoubtedly exists one condemning it and visa versa. A nutritional positive or negative can probably be found concerning any food under certain conditions and circumstances. For example, if you were to eat nothing else but great quantities of carrots, a generally agreed upon healthful food, all day, every day, soon enough, you'd be dead. But when we reach a point where certain studies, be they nutrition or exercise-oriented, are so blatantly skewed in the direction to benefit no one other than those cashing in while doing harm to those most in need, we are then careening wildly down a highway with ambiguous and confusing road signs.

When it comes to food studies, science has a bad habit of zeroing in on one particular nutrient that's been taken out of context and examining it in a singular fashion. For example, antioxidant vitamins E and C and beta carotene occur in a variety of foods. They were celebrated as marvel cures for everything from the common cold to heart disease and cancer by some in the scientific community. It didn't take long for vitamin and health food manufacturers to hear the good news and begin producing these vitamins with great alacrity. Utilizing their army of advertisers, the vitamin producers, not wanting to miss out on a big payday, began singing the praises of the miracle vitamins. This is how the propaganda machine, driven by the media, manipulates the public to purchase the next surefire, no doubt about it, can't miss health discovery. If something is loudly repeated enough times, it becomes "the truth," especially if the public accepts the teller as a credible source of information.

The vitamin manufacturers, promoters and media are all winners in this case, making money on the backs of unsuspecting consumers. The public loses as it spends money on trendy health discoveries while their health gets no better. These vitamin pills usually contain exceedingly high percentages of the recommended daily dosage. Many are 1,000% + of the recommended minimum amount. Some supplements have no daily recommended amount because scientists simply don't know what that amount should be. Science too often fails to realize that when a nutrient is taken out of context and consumed in isolated, concentrated doses, it may not have the same effect as eating the whole food containing that specific nutrient. Foods contain dozens of nutrients and chemicals that interact with one another in ways that science is not even close to figuring out yet.

Even if a study of a specific nutrient were held to the highest moral and ethical standards, the fact remains that conclusions reached regarding this nutritive substance would be suspect because of its isolation. Missing from the research would be the results of how it reacts in the presence of the materials making up the whole food. It may be a case where the vitamin still exhibits the same properties, whether alone or as part of the whole food. But we don't know that to be a fact if it's only studied alone. As it happens, if it were analyzed within the frame of reference of the whole food, we would still have no way of knowing if the vitamin behaves the way it does because of its interactions with the known constituents of the whole food or as a result of the presence of yet undiscovered components and their properties contained within the whole food. Science doesn't have all the answers.

Obviously, it's good for business when a company's product is cast in a positive light. Scientists who are paid by a particular company to study a product made by that company will try to find something positive to report about the food being studied, no matter how obscure or insignificant that positive may be. Like everyone else, they want to keep their jobs. They are beholden to those paying them. This is not to suggest that they are blatantly lying about food because they don't have to. All that a researcher needs to do is focus on and talk up a possible benefit, even if twisted logic has to be utilized while downplaying or simply making no mention of the negatives.

A good example of this behavior can be seen in a product I mentioned earlier, breakfast cereals. The overwhelming majority of cereals on the market today are, to put it bluntly, junk food. And I'm being liberal with my use of the word "food." They are nothing more than refined grains suffused with refined sugar, other sweeteners, salt, artificial coloring agents and other chemicals. Even the "better" ones are made up of at least some of these substandard ingredients, which have no place in a healthful diet. But what if we were to take one of these cereals with all their lousy ingredients and add some vitamins, minerals and/or a bit of whole grain? Well, now we would have created part of a nutritious breakfast. How? Simple, because scientific studies have shown that a diet containing _____ (fill in the blank with the latest magic bullet) has been shown to lower, raise, improve, eliminate, prevent, reverse _____ (fill in the blank with the latest medical condition). It comes down to how the findings are reported and interpreted. The glass may be half-empty, but it's also half-full.

Most consumers rely solely on taste when purchasing food. Many delude themselves into believing that they're doing something beneficial by purchasing the typically salty, sugary and fatty foods that they're convinced have been transformed into health foods due to the addition of a trendy vitamin, grain or other hyped ingredient. They don't have to give up the taste of sugar, salt or fat and can justify the consumption of these products because scientific studies have shown that the latest fashionable ingredient has health benefits. Thousands of these inferior products exist and continue to be manufactured because of consumer demand rooted in ignorance and wishful thinking. You may think you can have your cake and eat it too, but the unvarnished truth is that you can't. The people who realize and accept this reality are the ones who stand a good chance of improving their health. Those who don't are destined to continue running in place like the hamster on the wheel.

Science has provided humanity with countless life-enhancing and life-saving discoveries in the nutrition field. Without good scientific research, we wouldn't know that vegans generally need to take a B12 supplement, that vitamins E and A are fat soluble and stored in the body and if you take too much E and/or A, you can overdose. Without science, we wouldn't know that vitamin D regulates the blood's phosphorus and calcium levels and is needed for bone growth. We wouldn't be aware that a deficiency in vitamin A causes night blindness or that a lack of folic acid can cause anemia and miscarriages in pregnant women. We would be unaware that scurvy is caused by a vitamin C deficiency, nor would we be enlightened to the myriad of important nutritional, fitness and overall health discoveries as a result of scientific research. The research and studies continue, and that's a good thing. Just bear in mind the other side of science.

11

Medical Profession

Being a doctor, nurse or other healthcare professional is a noble calling. Helping to heal the sick and injured is indeed an occupation that deserves our respect and admiration. I'm certain nearly all of us have suffered one malady or another, visited a doctor and been cured or at least had our condition mitigated. The problem is that medical people usually excel at diagnosing and correcting diseases but aren't very well-schooled in the practice of preventing them in the first place.

Once we get past genetics, environment and luck, the prevention of illness and injury is predicated upon lifestyle. An unhealthful lifestyle usually equates to an unhealthy person. A healthful lifestyle is most often associated with a healthy person. For the indecisive among us, a moderately healthful way of life usually results in an average, moderately healthy person. It's not exactly a ringing endorsement for moderation. As I mentioned, there are always aberrations, but I don't think a reasonable individual would disagree with my overall conclusions about lifestyle. Two of the main components of a healthful lifestyle are exercise and proper nutrition.

As I reflect upon my personal medical history, it's profoundly and disturbingly clear that most doctors, nurses and other professional health practitioners that I've visited throughout my life have had very little to offer by way of helpful nutrition and exercise advice. Medical professionals are a microcosm of society, and as such, most of them are, in the best-case scenario, overweight and, at worst, obese. We're already familiar with all the illnesses brought about or exacerbated by being overweight and obese, but these facts take on a new dimension when you walk into a medical facility and are greeted by an overwhelming majority of fat, unhealthy-looking doctors and nurses. It does little to inspire or instill a sense of confidence in a patient. Based on the fact that medicine is their chosen profession, shouldn't they at least look like they care about their own well-being? These are people we hold to a higher standard. They have first hand knowledge of what becomes of a human body if it's not properly maintained.

Seeing nurses on break and smoking outside a medical building is something that still occurs. I've witnessed doctors with boxed donuts and cans of soda on their office desks. I've heard doctors tell a cancer patient to drink commercially available, yet nutritionally horrendous, energy drinks hoping that the patient can regain body weight. A nutritionally astute person wouldn't suggest a healthy person consume these energy drinks, let alone a cancer patient. Unfortunately, this is the advice that some doctors give to their patients, even though there are much better homemade alternatives available. I find it fascinating as I think back to numerous doctor's appointments and realize how often I've given them eating and exercise advice as they were examining me. This is not to say that I have their medical knowledge because I don't. Rather, it's to shed a bit of light on how much the medical profession does not know about nutrition, exercise and the importance each plays in preventing disease and injury.

If you listen, watch or read the news on a regular basis, chances are that you're aware of the deadliest diseases in America: heart disease, cancer, high blood pressure, stroke and diabetes. You also know that many, if not most, of these illnesses can be traced back to a poor diet and lack of proper exercise. This is not recent news. The warnings about preventable diseases and how they relate to diet and exercise have been sounded continually for decades. Yet, despite this knowledge, most doctors receive only the barest minimum nutrition instruction when they attend medical school. This is also common knowledge. I can only surmise that if there is a paucity of nutritional instruction given to doctors in training, even the most rudimentary form of exercise information as it relates to disease prevention must be all but nonexistent.

Over the years, I've had many out-of-shape and overweight doctors compliment me on my overall health and advise me to keep doing "whatever" it is I'm doing. They've been clueless as to why I'm not like the majority of their patients. This is discouraging for the general public because people go to doctors for answers and solutions. Their lack of knowledge about both food and exercise as medicine due to inadequate or nonexistent curriculum is incredible if you stop and think about all the education and training required for one to become a medical doctor. A clear case of "Physician heal thyself."

Years ago I was undergoing a routine annual physical examination. As the doctor and I were sitting in her office going over the results, she asked me how I generally felt about my overall health. I took the opportunity to complain about some soreness in my right knee and some discomfort in my left elbow. She, being a workout person and healthful eater, as she had informed me during our conversation and appearing to be a conditioned athlete, chuckled at my complaints of joint soreness. Not that the doctor dismissed them out of hand. On the contrary, my concerns were thoroughly discussed. She smiled as she told me that she wished that she had more patients with injuries due to exercise overuse than patients who underused their bodies and augmented this lack of movement by consuming disease-promoting food. She added that nothing is perfect, the positives far outweighed the negatives for my chosen way of living. The doctor further stated that it was extremely unlikely that my complaints would be the death of me, unlike the majority of her patients whose complaints would more than likely kill them. This doctor also instructed me to keep doing exactly what I was doing, not "whatever" I was doing. She knew precisely what I was doing because she was doing the same thing. This was the most beneficial and rewarding conversation I've ever had with a doctor. Sadly, she was the only doctor I've met who understood and applied her knowledge. I suppose there are others out there, but they are few and far between.

12

Pharmaceutical Industry

Figuring out the pharmaceutical industry doesn't entail a great deal of sleuthing. Does anyone out there actually believe that this multibillion-dollar-per-year earnings behemoth actually cares about your well-being? What this industry cares about is you when you're unhealthy. To put a finer point on this statement, big pharma cares about getting your money when you're unwell. The more unhealthy you are, the more of their products you'll buy. The more pills, syrups, powders and other drugs they can sell you, guarantees that their wealth and that of their stockholders will grow. These companies are publicly held and exist for the primary purpose of making profits and meeting Wall Street expectations. They are first beholden to their shareholders. It's all quite ugly but also quite legal and their prerogative. Remember, this is the United States of America, where capitalism rules, and profit comes before people.

I realize that the research and development of new drugs is an expensive proposition. Businesses exist to make money, which I fully understand and agree with. But when you reach a point where certain life-sustaining medications are so outrageously priced, well beyond the means of what the average person can afford, then there exists a moral and ethical problem. People shouldn't have to choose between paying their rent and purchasing medication when they are in dire need.

For at least the last few decades, the pharmaceutical giants have employed a brilliant strategy. During this time, as Americans have grown fatter and sicker, big pharma has pushed a campaign that doesn't promote cures for diseases, but instead it focuses on how people can live with and manage their afflictions. Granted, there are some conditions that cannot be truly cured and the unfortunate patients have no choice but to live with them as best as possible. If medications exist that will at least alleviate the suffering of people, this is without doubt a positive. But when the public is encouraged to live with and manage diseases that are mostly preventable, self-inflicted and often reversible, then we are dealing with a situation so twisted as to defy any logical thought.

Pharmaceutical America, in unofficial concert with the rest of the enablers, continues to promote the implied message that most people want to hear. The message is that we can persist with our current dietary habits, the very habits responsible for the diseases we presently endure.

We needn't fear that these diseases will run amuck in our bodies because the ailments will be managed by the variety of medications churned out by the pharmaceutical industrial complex.

We live in a country where being overweight and unfit are normal. We engage in all the behaviors that have caused most of the population to arrive at this precarious state of health. These behaviors are enthusiastically embraced and encouraged, and it's plain to see that there's very little will or desire among the populace for meaningful and significant change. Why exercise when it's so sweaty, uncomfortable and boring? Exercise is for obsessive, narcissistic types. Who wants to eat unpalatable, healthful food? People don't want vegetables, nuts, fruits, seeds, legumes and whole grains. They want to chow down on burgers, bacon, hotdogs, steak, fried chicken, chips, ice cream, refined-flour bread and pasta, cheesy pizza and the like. Just about any combination of salt, sugar and fat will temporarily sate America's voracious appetite for food that fosters disease. In addition to this problem, the consumption of alcohol, soda, energy drinks and coffee gives the appearance that we are a very thirsty nation, lacking in vitality and unable to deal with reality.

Subliminally, the pharmaceuticals are saying that we should eat, drink and be merry. No need to change anything. Keep on enjoying. If all this merriment causes you an illness, it can easily be managed with drugs. Go ahead. No need to deny yourself the pleasures of life. If you've got a problem, we've got a drug.

A while back, a plump acquaintance told me that his overall cholesterol number was a whopping 360 and that he also suffered from hypertension. This individual actually exercised, albeit sporadically and incorrectly and yet, much to his surprise, he gained more weight. He announced to me with a great deal of pride that he worked out regularly. He also informed me that he was taking various medications to keep his elevated cholesterol and high blood pressure within acceptable parameters so that he could eat whatever he wanted. His idea of a healthful way of life was to exercise, medicate himself and eat anything he desired. On several occasions he offered that if you couldn't eat as much of anything you craved, then there was no point to life. That was his wellness plan. Sadly, I've discovered through my experiences that his philosophy is not uncommon. He told me that I was crazy for doing what I did when all he had to do was ingest his prescribed medications and not change a thing in his life.

All medications have potential side effects, a fact that doesn't appear to be diminishing the desire of the masses for foods that encourage the sicknesses that, in turn, require the medications. Nothing like having a disease to concern yourself with and compounding that stress with potentially causing more medical issues by taking the very drugs that are supposed to be maintaining some sort of healthful equilibrium. This indifference regarding medications, whether prescription or over-the-counter, can have serious health consequences for the individual being medicated. The situation can readily become a good news/bad news scenario. The good news is that the medication you're taking is managing your high cholesterol, but the bad news is that you're suffering from headaches, diarrhea and muscle weakness.

The bottom line is that you cannot simply continue abusing yourself while looking to the pharmaceutical gods to provide a miracle drug so that you may continue to abuse yourself. These drug lords depend on your weaknesses and use them to their formidable advantage as a way to keep the money rolling in. You need to decide if you're comfortable with that or if a radical change of behaviors on your part is in order.

13

Celebrities And Wellness

We are a culture that worships youth, money and celebrity, though not necessarily in that order. Many of us have anointed the usual celebrities as experts in the field of fitness and nutrition. To be clear, I'm not referring to those folks who are celebrities as a result of being experts in the field of fitness and nutrition but to the individuals we consecrate as such, despite the fact that they aren't experts in this field. I'm referencing the typical array of professional athletes, models, actors, TV chefs, talk show hosts and entertainers. As with everyone else I've mentioned, these people are as human as we are. They have strengths and weaknesses. Too many of us automatically assume that they're health gurus for no reason other than the fact that they're wealthy and famous. Celebrity status alone is a pretty flimsy requirement for becoming a health and fitness expert. As far as their habits are concerned, celebrities are an exemplification of the greater society, and while it's obvious they possess fame and much greater wealth than the rest of us, they are no more than that.

I'm in no way criticizing each one's talents in his or her respective vocation. As a matter of fact, I'm not criticizing celebrities at all. They're as entitled to earn a living as are the rest of us. If corporations dealing with any of the wide variety of products under the health and fitness umbrella wish to pay the rich and famous for testimonials, which have nothing to do with their occupations, that's their business. What I find simultaneously curious, silly and obsequious is the way so many of us hang on to every word a famous person utters when it comes to, in this specific example, a health and fitness topic, despite the fact that the celebs don't manage their wellness any better or worse than do the unwashed masses.

Athletes who stay in good condition for the rest of their lives once they retire are in the minority. Most gain unhealthful weight. There's no need to mention names here if you watch sports. Models are traditionally known for starving themselves. Nothing healthful about that. However, there does seem to be a movement afoot to curtail that practice, which is good news. There's no argument here that chefs on TV cook up some mighty tasty-looking dishes. Remember that just because something looks and tastes good doesn't mean it's good for you. Many TV chefs boast about their healthful recipes. Depends on your definition of healthful. If your idea of what constitutes healthful coincides with that of the TV chef, have at it. Mostly, what I see on TV cooking shows is salt, sugar, butter, oils, refined flour and meat. These ingredients don't live up to my standard of what's healthful, nor should they live up to yours if your health is the priority. The priority of actors is their art. How many of these people have you seen transform their bodies, depending on the character they are portraying, from thin to fat to muscular to everything in between? Unless the individual was a poor physical specimen, to begin with, then suddenly trained him or herself into top condition and maintained it for life, these bodyweight gains and losses wreak havoc on the system. Again, bad for one's health. For the most part, celebrities whose livelihoods depend on the very bodies they inhabit, mostly athletes and models, have trainers, nutritionists and wide-ranging support teams to keep their bodies in top form while they enjoy their careers. Basically, they stay in shape because it's their responsibility as a part of their job, not because they prioritize their health and fitness. This is the reason so many of them decline physically when they retire.

As far as TV talk show hosts go, when it comes to dispensing nutrition, fitness and weight loss information, again, I find it fascinating that so many are riveted by the messages being put forth by these famous individuals. Fame has not immunized many of them from continuing to struggle with their own weight issues. Perhaps it's nothing more than a type of commiseration. I don't know.

Athletes need to possess the required levels of strength, speed, power, quickness and many other nuanced abilities in order to stay in the game. They need to be relatively fit and healthy. Something to bear in mind is that, unlike athletes, the "beautiful people" need only appear to be in fine condition. Many are what I often refer to as superficially healthy. They look great on the outside, but most maintain acceptable weight through calorie counting, not by leading healthful lives. We've all heard and read many interviews where young svelte actors and other entertainers were asked how they stay in such great condition. Translation, how they keep looking good. Looking good does not necessarily equate to being in great condition, especially if you're polluting your insides.

Many of these rich and famous personalities have responded to an interviewer's question regarding their impressive appearance with such illuminating answers as, "Oh, I eat what I want. I'm just lucky, I guess." or "I hate to exercise. I'm simply blessed." or "I merely eat smaller portions of everything. I don't deny myself at all." When we account for the facelifts, tucks, dermatological skin peels, implants, liposuction and collagen injections, it becomes blatantly apparent that we are no longer discussing health at this juncture. We're talking about a beautiful, shiny Lamborghini parked at the curb, but under the hood, the engine has seized.

The main takeaway here is that we do ourselves a disservice when we compare ourselves physically to this group of people. Don't look to Hollywood, with its silly array of fad diets, weight loss techniques and secrets, for help. You may lose weight in the short term, but you'd be far better off thinking about health, not simply calories and pounds. In the long term, following the advice of these people will once again cause you to waste your precious time and money, yet bring you nothing but failure and disappointment. When you take control of your health via proper nutrition and exercise, improving yourself to the point where you are the best that you can be, given your genetic potential, then you have achieved success.

14

Media

By media, I'm primarily referring to all print, electronic and digital embodiments, although other forms exist. The media is a double-edged sword. On the one hand, a free and open news media reports whatever it wishes without fear of reprisal from authoritarian governments. This benefits the country along with its citizens. As long as the reporting doesn't constitute slander, the media is free to report what it considers newsworthy. A good independent news media keeps us informed about events and occurrences of which we would otherwise be ignorant. It's a given that what is reported at times may cause us to disagree as to what qualifies as news. However, the overall knowledge we gain from the information provided is substantially empowering. Reports of new scientific discoveries, political corruption, medical news, dangerous impending weather systems, natural disasters, traffic delays, local events and even some entertainment news enhance both the quality and efficiency of our daily lives.

The other edge of the media sword is its dull edge. The media and news reporting have become part of the entertainment industry. Although examples of this can be seen across the bulk of news reporting platforms, it's most obvious on network and cable TV. It's as if the producers believe we are all suffering from attention deficit disorder (ADD). It's a hodgepodge of music, color and flash, all presented in a slick fashion. Many TV news anchors could hold second jobs as models. They grace our screens with their attractiveness, giggling and joking with one another on air, only to seamlessly segue to the solemn news-face that is required for the reporting of a tragic story. Televised news today is routinely sensationalized, replete with distracting quick camerawork, teasers and too many inane accounts of happenings that one would be hard-pressed to qualify as notable.

Gone are the days of Walter Cronkite, Chet Huntley, David Brinkley, Roger Mudd, John Chancellor and Howard K. Smith. These iconic journalists and TV news presenters from a different period in our country's history, along with others, reported the cold, dry facts—what a news report should be. No editorializing for them. That's what editorials are for. There was certainly no chance of catching any one of these gentlemen in Bermuda shorts while doing a piece at an Independence Day block party and barbecue, reporting what was on the menu, then sampling same and gushing at the deliciousness of it all while the studio team provided equally silly and unnewsworthy commentary.

In bygone days when the news was news, the presenters didn't tell the audience to wear a hat and gloves on cold winter days, nor did they feel compelled to remind us to wear sun protection during the summer. Today we hear these same reminders from TV news people, over and over again and season after season. These reminders, along with similar cues, are what our mothers are supposed to do. This is yet another clear example of the dumbing down of our society. If we require the media for instructions on seasonal modes of dress, then our chances of survival as a species are surely more diminished.

The media is a very powerful force in America today. It has a tremendous influence on the behaviors of the population, including what we wear, drive, do for entertainment, how we rear our children and unquestionably what we eat and drink. One needs to be equipped with confidence and a strongly developed sense of self in order to deflect the unyielding media bombardment of information we are subjected to twenty-four hours a day, every day. From the behaviors I've observed and conversations I've heard, I'd say that a great number of people don't possess a strong sense of self and suffer from varying degrees and types of insecurities. However, I don't believe most would admit to this human frailty because they are attempting to promote and maintain an image of self-assurance.

Another of the many things the masses have in common is the emotional inability to stand alone. Most feel a need to behave in a manner that falls in line with what is socially accepted and embraced. The refrains, "Everybody is doing it" and "Keeping up with the Joneses" come to mind. Combine this attitude with insecurity, and it follows that the preponderance of our nation's inhabitants are not doers but are constantly being done to, socially speaking. This is a boon for the media and plays right into their hands. It's also a godsend for those using the media as instruments to spread their respective agendas. As a result, the media can basically mold and manipulate you into behaving in ways that no confident, rational, critically thinking human would consider. The general message that providers of food and drink have foisted upon the public through the use of media outlets cuts across all racial, religious, ethnic, gender-specific, generational, educational and socioeconomic boundaries. At its most basic, the message can be encapsulated in the idea that eating and drinking are fun pastimes. This message has been sewn into the very fabric of our culture since the dawn of societal development and recorded history. As technology has improved over the ages, it has been easier to spread the message. Today this message has become an avalanche of enabling and encouraging commentary to eat and drink like never before. Unfit, overweight people can be found in all the aforementioned societal groups. The message is powerful and obviously gets through to the vast majority of the populace. And at what cost? I'm not referring to the cost in dollars, although it's massive and creates its own set of societal problems, but to the cost of an individual's health.

The price is staggering when you consider that almost three-quarters of the American population is overweight. In a country of more than 330,000,000 inhabitants, that amounts to about 247,500,000 people. It's well known that there are approximately 25-30,000,000 diabetes sufferers and untold tens of millions more yet to be diagnosed who, if not outright diabetic, are pre-diabetic. Another well-known statistic is that heart disease kills anywhere from 500,000 to 600,000 people in the United States each year. Most of these deaths are easily preventable because they are more often than not attributable to lifestyle.

Despite all this alarming news, we continue to focus on individual diseases that, while devastating to the sufferer, don't even come close to affecting the number of people who become sick and die due to our Western diet, lifestyle and attitude. It's true that the powers that be bring attention to illnesses such as heart disease, diabetes, certain cancers, stroke and hypertension. Yet their efforts to directly and in no uncertain terms attribute these maladies to unwise decisions by those afflicted are tepid and feckless. Also lacking is strong language to further drive home the point that most of these cases were preventable in the first place and, in many cases, reversible. It's the type of improvement in which nothing gets better.

People love symbolism because it makes them feel good about themselves. They embrace being part of a movement, believing they're doing their part in helping to find a solution for whichever health problem is currently trending. We hold pancake, sausage, bacon and egg breakfasts at our local community centers, houses of worship and volunteer firehouses to raise money to find a cure for heart disease. What's next, wine-tasting affairs to raise money to find a cure for alcoholism? Does no one see the irony and utter stupidity in these behaviors, or are these facts simply ignored? The media is front and center promoting these feel-good activities. Unfortunately, there are no races for curing overweight, no walks to combat lousy food choices and no potluck dinners to assist the unfit. The reason for this is that these conditions and habits are overwhelmingly normal, not something to be cured.

There doesn't exist a pink ribbon pin, little red dress pin or any type of awareness pin or silicone awareness bracelet announcing to the world that we are in solidarity in our battle against "fat and unfit due to eating bad food." When the problem is even considered, we rail against the specific disease, sound the alarm and engage in cultural hand-wringing. The familiar commissions, committees and subcommittees are formed, dates are set for more meetings and facts and figures are analyzed and reanalyzed. There is also a great deal of talking, at which these groups excel. The media assures us the problem is being addressed, but in the end, it's business as usual.

Another aspect stemming from the dull side of the media's double-edged sword is the marginalization of a minority group. This is no minority in the traditional sense of the word or what one usually expects when the word is invoked. Most often, it is mentioned only when its members are being ridiculed by the media in a movie, TV show, book, magazine article, advertisement or by the public at large. The main characteristic uniting the people in this underrepresented group is that they live like they care. This is not unlike the pernicious messages encouraging self-destructive behaviors emanating from the media, cutting across all the boundaries I mentioned earlier. The desire to embrace health and fitness while ignoring all the noise also cuts across those boundaries, albeit to a much lesser extent. It's quite clear that healthful living does not have the same panache as the messages promoting self-abuse. Yet, the health-positive message is reaching some people which does provide a spark of optimism for a portion of our species. I would argue that the ideas of Charles Darwin and Alfred Russel Wallace may be at work here, natural selection through "survival of the fittest." Once that portion of the population succeeds in killing itself off as a result of choices made that prove to be inconsistent with long-term survival, humanity will evolve into a far more healthy and intelligent primate.

Although dispersed far and wide, the marginalized group's constituents remain united through a powerful will to be the best versions of themselves. This is despite the fact that members of the group are most often painted by the loudest parts of the media as being extremists, fanatics and bereft of all of life's pleasures. Pleasures that include caffeine, alcohol, soda, fast food, junk food and all the other toxic substances I mentioned earlier, which humans ingest in their never-ending quest for fun. The ridicule vacillates between overt and subtle but is present nonetheless. Compounding this with a general distaste and avoidance of meaningful exercise by mainstream citizens and incited by aspects of the media, it's no wonder the derisive term "health nut" has burgeoned throughout the cultural vernacular. What kind of label are we then to bestow on those who insist on harming the only body they will ever inhabit? Deacons of decrepitude, wizards of weakness, haters of health, faithfully unfit and desirers of disease are a few that spring to mind. Perhaps the best adjective that can be used to describe those champions of self-inflicted disease is "normal," for the normal far outnumber the "health nuts."

While the normal continue to rush with reckless abandon toward unnecessary disease and early death, convinced that they're having fun along the way, those who live like they care will persist in doing just that. For these people, the content coming from the media is simply an irritating distraction. Those who embrace health and fitness to the highest level possible will carry on with proper exercise, enjoy plant-based diets and eschew alcohol, caffeine, soda and processed pseudo foods. They, unlike their unwise brethren, will have no need for medications and unending medical appointments for illnesses they have brought upon themselves. When they step out of the shower, those who embrace health will be content with their mirrored reflection, not due to vanity, although there is nothing wrong with pride in a job well done, but, because they have the peace of mind of knowing that they are doing the absolute best they can with what they were given. At each year's annual physical, barring an event beyond their control, they'll be rewarded with a clean bill of health. There's also a very good chance that the doctor will ask these people what they're doing to remain so fit and healthy.

Yes, the media has greatly contributed to the concept that those inhabiting the marginalized group are weird, obsessive, narcissistic, compulsive, extreme, abnormal and, of course, health nuts. The media is absolutely correct about one thing for sure, this group is definitely not normal. Normal is vastly overrated and is what most children, without the benefit of life experiences, want to be. A prudent adult outgrows the silly notions and desires of a guileless child unless he doesn't. When he doesn't, that lack of development can be readily seen in the adult version.

Examples of the media perpetuating the negative stereotype of people who truly take care of their health abound in novels, cinema, advertisements, music, magazines and much more. I'm well aware that the media also touches upon healthful subject matter. However, as previously discussed, my mission is to wake you from your torpor to enlighten you of the reality that helpful content is crushed by noxious content. I suppose it's just not cool to treasure your health. The edgy, hip people, especially in our youth-centric culture, are usually portrayed as partiers, drinkers of alcohol, smokers, vapers, recreational drug users, consumers of all manner of disease-promoting food, coffee drinkers, soda drinkers, energy drink gulpers and indulgers of any combination of these behaviors. Today, normal people in America, if not the world, undeniably demonstrate at least a few of these tendencies, especially where food and drink are concerned. These normal people are mostly of the overweight unfit variety but also include the skinny unfit. No rational, reasonably intelligent human should aspire to be normal, to be average, as I've described the term. The wiser course for all concerned is to shoot for something better in order to improve. Once we reach some semblance of adulthood, it should be evident that if you do what everyone else is doing, you're going to wind up like everyone else.

On this planet where profits come before people, the media is primarily about making money, especially from advertiser dollars. There is nothing illegal about this. However, don't delude yourself into thinking that this ubiquitous communication apparatus truly cares about your health. The broadcast networks care about ratings first because ratings equal advertisers, and advertisers equal more revenue for the networks. Newspapers, magazines and social media sites all sell ad space to produce further profits. Did you ever stop and think how incongruent it is to be watching a news report about the terrible worldwide obesity epidemic when what immediately follows is a commercial for Burger King, Wendy's, McDonald's, Pizza Hut, Kentucky Fried Chicken, Taco Bell, Dunkin', Starbucks, Budweiser and on and on? Don't you find the mixed message a little screwy? It's stupefying to be watching a TV news reporter informing the audience about a body-fat related health issue such as heart disease, hypertension or diabetes, when suddenly, without skipping a beat, the very next segment is a reporter at some restaurant showing us how the chef prepares those "sinful yet delectable" holiday cakes, cookies and treats. Back at the studio, the anchors are so into it they can't wait to chime in with ridiculous comments of approval while informing us how they, too, will be indulging in these treats during the holidays. It's normal, right?

Mixed media messages are prolific. Think about standing in a grocery store checkout aisle. Look around at all the candy and other junk food strategically placed in the location just before you pay for your purchases and exit the store. It's the final temptation of the shopper. What else do you see sharing the racks in this area? Of course, the magazines. Celebrity magazines are mainstays so we can keep up with the exploits of the rich and famous. Magazines geared towards beautifying our homes can usually be found along with the rags announcing that Elvis is alive and living with an extraterrestrial in Ashtabula. In addition to the garbage masquerading as something we should eat and the mostly lowbrow publications, the reading material that predominates are the periodicals purposely geared toward women for obvious reasons. Everyone knows that it's women who are likeliest to diet. What better way to exploit this knowledge than with an endless stream of articles on easy and fun weight loss tips? While some of these glossies include relatively helpful articles now and again, most do a great disservice to women. It's bewildering how anyone can take these magazines seriously when the headlines, almost universally pertaining to weight loss and slimming down, make proclamations such as "The Miracle Weight Loss Secret Revealed," "Blast Fat Away in 30 Minutes!," "Hidden Fat Traps," "Burn Fat With This Snack," "Get Slim For Good," "Lose 10 Pounds Fast Without The Cravings," "Flat Tummy, Slim Legs & Tight Tush In One Easy Workout!," "Get Your Body Beach Ready Fast," "Eat This To Drop Those Extra Pounds," "Free Yourself From Emotional Eating," "Drop A Dress Size In Minutes" and "The Workout That Melts Fat Away." It would be terrific if any of these declarations and their accompanying articles were completely true. The first problem is they aren't. The second problem arises when these periodicals, in an attempt to evoke a feeling of health and fitness with blaring cover headlines similar to these, share equal space on these very same covers with headlines such as "Sinfully Delicious Chocolate Cake For Chocolate Lovers," "Cookie Cravers Recipes," "Frightfully Dangerous Halloween Cupcakes," "Cure Depression—Eat Christmas Cookies!," "Mouthwatering Ham Recipes For Easter," "Tasty Corned Beef & Cabbage For St. Patrick's Day," "Sweet Treats For Your Valentine," "Take Thanksgiving To The Next Level With These Irresistible Desserts," "Fire Up Your Grill For The Best Burgers & Hotdogs This 4th," "Score A Touchdown With Winning Super Bowl Chow," "Easy Cheesy Pasta," "Creamy Dips For Your Favorite Chips," "Chunky Cheese And Bacon Dressing To Liven Up Any Salad" and "Magnificent Muffins In Minutes."

Each of these magazines employs the classic example of playing both sides, trying to be all things to all people. This sort of policy is impossible. Every one of them casts the widest net in order to garner as many reader dollars as possible—a seemingly smart business move but a demonstrable model for schizophrenic advertising if ever there was one. It's another example of confusing people when they are desperately searching for guidance. The publications show themselves for what they are to an astute observer by failing to display a strength of conviction concerning health and fitness because they lack that conviction..

A simple glance of the recipes reveals the usual suspects: added sugar, added salt, artificial coloring agents, saturated and hydrogenated fats, nitrite and nitrate-infused deli meats, heart-clogging cheeses and creams, processed worthless white flour, dairy, animal products and difficult-to-pronounce chemicals. These items don't appear on the menus of the minority of people who are absolutely unapologetically serious about their health and fitness unless they are starving to death without any alternative.

In September 2009, I happened to hear a profoundly foolish commercial broadcast by a Binghamton, New York, FM radio station. Remembering the date was easy because I found the advertisement so outlandish. I immediately took notes and filed them away where I keep such things for potential future use. The ad's purpose was to encourage listeners to attend a local fundraiser benefiting Alzheimer's disease research, an incontrovertible worthy cause. Dismally, the commercial quickly spiraled downward, losing all credibility as the manic announcer implored his audience to join others at this function, where they could all "eat wings and drink soda and beer!" This is akin to my previous example of pancake and sausage socials to raise money for funding heart disease research. No need to elaborate further, as my point is painfully obvious.

Countless similar and related examples, fueled by media, abound every day if we simply take the time to pay attention. People can choose to have a resigned temperament in the face of this relentless assault on our collective intelligence. They can succumb and join the party to preventable demise or choose to be resilient by adhering to an unyielding conviction regarding health. The media is like a high-priced prostitute in that it will do whatever you desire if the price is right. It seems as if a day can't go by without some sort of report, be it print or electronic, referencing the state of America's persistently bulging waistline. Placing financial gains first, they admonish, "America, you're fat!" and in the next breath, "Hey, let's all go to McDonald's for fries and a shake." America is a skinny-worshipping culture of mostly fat and unfit people. These people are encouraged by the media to eat all manner of detrimental food. Simultaneously, the media offers two distinct messages. First, it alerts the people about the dangers of being overweight, as a result of eating detrimental food. Then, it encourages them to eat this very same food. If anyone sees a problem here, please raise your hand. Manipulation through propaganda runs rampant across America.

15

Illusion

There exist entire industries built on the promise that they will help you to improve your looks. On its surface, there's nothing wrong with this, and moreover, I would argue that a greater number of people, at least superficially, wish to look their best most of the time. Therefore, these industries generally provide a service that is in demand. It's well known that depending on an individual's body type, skin tone and hair color, one's appearance can be enhanced or diminished depending on clothing and hairstyle choices. This seems logical.

Let's explore this subject of appearance from another perspective. The intention of so many people to not simply want to look their best but to create an illusion completely apart from their true selves is compelling. Again, women seem to be most often targeted, but by no means do all men escape exploitation. The subgroups that usually acquiesce to suggestive advertising are young, impressionable women, overweight women and women in what is commonly referred to as middle age. What is one to make of the scuba suit-like undergarments that squish your fat and flatten it out in an attempt to make you appear thinner? Appear, is the operative word here. And what of the creams that magically make wrinkles disappear to help you achieve that youthful glow once again? You can apply a countless array of lotions that promise to melt away fat and cellulite. Want to give a taller impression? Wear vertically striped outfits and/or wear high-heeled shoes to pull off that pretense. Men going gray can color their hair and beards. Nothing like seeing a man who is obviously on the slippery slope side of the mountain of life with shoe polish black hair. Going bald? No problem, a nice hairpiece will do the trick because they're always so convincing. Greater aspirations? Then hair transplants might do the trick.

Think your eyelashes are lacking? Don't be concerned—just slap on a pair of the false variety. You can shave off your real eyebrows and instead have artificial ones drawn, tattooed, glued or microbladed in their place for that natural look. Another option is to have these procedures done in conjunction with your existing eyebrows, in essence, working around what you've got. Don't like the color of your eyes? You can purchase eye color-changing lenses. Really committed to changing your eye color? There's always the alternative of eye color-change surgery. Call me a sissy, but this one scares the hell out of me, and I don't recommend it. Then again, if my important parts and pieces are functioning well, I tend to adhere to the old adage, "If it ain't broke, don't fix it." Change of eye color does not rate very high on the list of improvements I believe one needs to focus on.

Women's breasts never fall out of fashion as an area of concern. If you're unhappy that yours are too small, there's always the padded brasier. For the mature, well-endowed among our female population on whom gravity has taken its toll, who wish to recapture, at least the youthful aspect of a high, firm bosom, upthrust bras will provide the desired look. Those seriously devoted to structural change can have small breasts enlarged or large breasts reduced through surgical procedures.

Throughout the years, the concept of what qualifies as the quintessential female backside has changed. The sought-after and accepted look at present is big and round. Once again we find culture at work dictating what the masses are expected to praise. Naturally, this caused consternation to many women concerning their unexpectedly less than desirable bottoms. Not to worry, for just as there appears to be an application for everything in the world on our digital devices, there also appears to be a fix for every body image problem, real or perceived, humankind can come up with. Butt implants anyone? It's difficult for me to wrap my head around the fact that this is a real thing. If this type of procedure is beyond your fortitudinous or your financial means, padded butt underwear is easily available for purchase. Take heed, men. You needn't feel disappointed that you'll be left out because padded undies are also available for you. Now, we can all rejoice as we mince about with our artificially enhanced rear ends, with the added knowledge that we are doing our part in conforming to the edicts of culture.

If you're a man or, for that matter, a woman who is so inclined and doesn't relish the idea of regular workouts to sculpt the body you desire, you can opt for muscle augmentation surgery. You can achieve the look of a bodybuilder without building your body. Liposuction procedures are very popular these days for those who prefer to continue eating as they do and would rather have excess fat vacuum-sucked through an incision made in their bodies.

In an effort to improve our image, we spend absurd amounts of money, time and sometimes pain on mostly smoke and mirror strategies. Either we go from the relatively benign, such as pedicures, manicures, makeup and intoxicating fragrances, or we vacillate between fatuous gimmicks and the previously described riskier approaches. Billions of dollars are allocated for techniques, gadgets, products and procedures to make us prettier and more handsome. In the end, none of it is real.

Good luck if you're catting about and enhanced to a state of irresistible attractiveness, presenting this illusion of yourself as a result of a combination of these strategies, and you happen to meet someone with whom you'd like to become intimate, and the feeling is reciprocal. What will you do when you need to discard some of the camouflage, all the illusionary paraphernalia and must stand naked before the object of your affection? I suppose you can do it in the dark, but that won't work for long. Eventually, the harsh reality of what you really look like will present itself. If you're fortunate, perhaps you'll both be resorting to illusionary tactics, laugh about it and live happily ever after. However, if you're the only one availing yourself to disguise techniques, there's a strong probability that your "conquest" will suddenly remember something very important that was forgotten and uncomfortably declare, "Gotta go, I'll call you!" as he or she beats a hasty exit. You, at this time, will be left crestfallen and embarrassed while pondering the wisdom or lack thereof, while considering that last double cheese, double dough, pepperoni, sausage pizza, deep-fried onion rings, garlic knots and Diet Coke.

Don't misconstrue what I'm saying. Many of the items and procedures I've described as illusionary techniques have their place, particularly with people who are stricken with cancer, for example, and have lost their hair due to chemotherapy. Some individuals may be dealing with afflictions that cause one type of disfigurement or another, causing them feelings of inadequacy and affecting their self-esteem. It's bad enough to be coping with a disease without further having to struggle with psychological trauma. Some of the modes of action I've portrayed are utilized by sick people who are in desperate need of a pick-me-up any way they can get it, considering what they are going through. I can't say I wouldn't take similar action in some cases.

But I'm not talking about, nor will I ever disparage, individuals who, through no fault of their own, are besieged by disease, disfigurement or mental incapacity. Genetics, medical conditions, accidents and a variety of other circumstances can claim any one of us at any time, thereby negatively impacting our appearances, if not our very lives. My ruminations are directly focused on the relatively healthy sector of the population. More specifically, the people who make up this majority group, were they to earnestly live in a manner conducive to health, would continue to inhabit their present chronological age, a factor beyond anyone's control, but would be biologically younger and look better than how society expects them to appear at their temporal number. If this were the case, there would be no need to engage in deceptive tactics to land a partner or to impress friends and colleagues. The takeaway here should be that if you spent half the time, money, dedication, commitment and focus on meaningful exercise, a healthful diet, eliminating alcohol, tobacco and caffeine, along with the assortment of other mental crutches, our culture has deemed indispensable, stopped complaining and searching for support groups for a solution to a problem that only you can solve, you'd find your insecurities greatly diminished. Logically speaking, how could they not be diminished if you're doing everything you possibly can to create the best, healthiest version of yourself, physically and emotionally?

Adults are often heard lecturing and urging children to live up to their potential. In most instances, this is clearly an exercise in hypocrisy since so few adults ever achieve this goal. We can't all be the best at a given skill or activity. That's life and must be accepted. What we can be is the best embodiment of ourselves. This is what success is. This is what freedom feels like. This is peace of mind.

You can only lie to yourself for so long by depending on smoke and mirrors to create a fictional version of yourself. I'm reminded of one of many porcine proverbs: "If you put makeup on a pig, what you then have is a pig wearing makeup." You'll never be this, so long as you're the best real you possible.

16

Culture And Tradition

The words *culture* and *tradition* are liberally cast about as if to imply that they only possess positive connotations. I'm as much in favor of these institutions as the next person, but only when engaging in the pragmatic aspects of each. When, as so often occurs, a facet of culture or tradition is at odds with the soundness of body and mind, general personal safety, the good of the environment, or the existence of the beneficial and benign lifeforms with which we share the earth, then these two words become nothing more than veiled excuses for unacceptable behaviors. Culture and tradition can be unquestionable sources of enhancement to the lives of people. They can also serve as undeniable justifications for foolish choices, harsh practices, totalitarian implementations, and repressive and deadly behaviors.

One need not conduct an in-depth analysis in order to discover examples of culture and tradition gone awry in ways extending from foolish to deadly. They exist in history and are easily seen today if we are willing to look. Slavery, religious/ethnic/racial and gender intolerance, including discrimination and extermination, ageism, supreme male domination over females, female genital mutilation, honor killings (usually of females), bull fighting, cock fighting and dog fighting, whaling, big game trophy hunting, college hazing rituals and innumerable habits and practices, whether dramatic or seemingly innocent, such as drinking beer and eating hot dogs at a ball game and eating ice cream, cake and candy at a birthday party, all have their genesis in culture and tradition. This fact does not make these practices right, good or healthful.

Culture and tradition are two of the more utilized words when it comes to eating and drinking behaviors. If you don't look at them critically, they're pleasant words that stimulate positive thoughts and feelings. However, if you're killing yourself as a result of them, they become malevolent. Health comes first, not culture and tradition. It makes no difference if your mother, grandmother, uncle, or whichever relative it may be is always cooking a traditional dish for a particular cultural celebration. If as a result of your research, education, and newfound commitment to health, you were to discover that your dear grandma's fare no longer fits within your dietary parameters, it would serve you well to politely decline the offering.

The chances of your relative handling this without insult or bad feelings are probably slim. I'm being realistic. This is not your problem to solve. This is where commitment and strength of conviction come into play. If asked why you're not partaking of the meal, you need to explain in a non-accusatory manner, the reasons for your decision. If she or he is typically insecure about these issues, you may have to go beyond simply explaining your health concerns and delve into reassurances of love and caring to express to the individual that it's nothing personal. Your dear relative can either accept this or not. That choice isn't yours. You've already chosen. It's as simple as that, so don't complicate the situation by worrying about hurt feelings.

Too often, we engage in absurd behaviors in the name of culture and tradition while unaware of the actual reasons why we are taking part in such conduct. Frequently, the reason serves no other purpose than to acknowledge that the inane habits are cultural and traditional. Few stop to think about the purpose or its consequences. Culture and tradition are poor inducements to consume food and drink that promote disease.

17

Excuses

Over the years, I've heard and continue to hear just about all the excuses people can invent for neglecting exercise, making poor food choices, and being habitually unfit. Often, the excuses arise from conversations I've had with unfit people seeking my advice about nutrition and exercise. During the conversations, rather than listening to my sound and honest counsel, these individuals immediately start to make excuses regarding their poor fitness and the reasons they can't act on my recommendations. It is fascinating to note that they believe their excuses are valid and original. Unfortunately, this belief system prevents them from improving their health, and it enables them to continue creating a problem for every nutrition and exercise solution I suggest. I also hear excuses among the self-debilitated people I encounter. These are the people who have ruined their own health based on poor lifestyle choices. When they ask me for nutritional guidance, they repeatedly interrupt my efforts, so they can inform me about their vast repository of nutritional acumen. If they know so much, why consult me? Perhaps, it's a case of expansive knowledge but poor application skills—I don't know.

The following is a comprehensive list of excuses I've endured throughout the years. Be honest with yourself; which one(s) have you employed?

1. "I don't have time to exercise."

The last time I checked, here on planet Earth, we all had and continue to have the same amount of time each day, 24 hours. The key here is what you choose to do with your time. You need to decide what's important. You can sit on the couch and watch TV while gorging on a bag of Cheetos and a six-pack of beer, or you can work out.

2. "Exercise takes too long."

Even if you've never exercised, you can work your way up to a very basic 30-minute daily session. If you're unwilling to devote 30 minutes out of your day, 5 to 7 days per week, to a routine that will indubitably benefit your health, then you just don't care enough because your priorities lie elsewhere.

3. "I'm in the office all day long."

You'll never hear a diseased, dying person with all manner of tubes and wires issuing forth from a neglected body and otherwise connected to life-sustaining machinery in the ICU at the hospital utter the words, "I knew I should have spent more time at the office."

4. "Exercise is hard."

Many things in life are hard, including having your sternum split open to grant the surgeon access to the heart you have so cavalierly destroyed. Having digits and limbs cleaved from your body due to rampant diabetes brought on by your insouciant choices of food and drink is hard. Most things worth striving for and achieving in this life are hard. Were this not the case, we'd all be successfully content millionaires, highly intelligent, with bodies like Greek gods and goddesses. The example and message you present to your children with this excuse is, "Don't try this. It's too hard."

5. "I'm too fat and embarrassed to go to the gym."

Granted, you're likely to find a smattering of fit and attractive people at a gym. This is no different an occurrence than in life's encounters outside the gym. If you are of the mind that all the members, except for you, are steroid-enabled examples of physical human perfection, trust me, they're not. Most of the specimens I've seen at gyms aren't remotely close to being in the condition required for entering, let alone winning, a body-beautiful contest any time soon.

6. "I can't afford a gym membership."

You don't need to train in a gym to improve your fitness. All you need is desire. If prison inmates in solitary confinement can develop their bodies in a tiny cell with nothing more than a bunk, table, toilet, and sink as equipment, each bolted to the floor, you'll need to rethink this one.

7. "I don't know which exercises to do."

Neither did I when I began. Be determined to find out. Tutorials, instructions, information, and tips on how to exercise abound. Read books and magazines. Watch TV exercise programs. We live in the digital age. Use your smartphone or computer for something useful like researching modes of exercise. Try exercise DVDs. Ask questions of acquaintances who are regular exercisers. As with anything else, you'll receive good, fair and poor information. Cherry pick. Filter out what doesn't work for you. Research and learn. Even if all else fails, walk. Don't stroll. Your first simple, brisk walk can be the beginning of an exercise program that changes your life. I'm pretty certain you know how to walk.

8. "Exercise is no fun."

Life is everything from fun to miserable. Life is life. Freshman algebra was no fun for most of us either, but we got through it anyway. When you begin to see the fruits of your labor manifested by the positive changes happening to your body, exercise, while still hard work, will be something you look forward to. You have to decide if it's more fun to be overweight, unfit, and barely able to walk or breathe.

Life is full of many things, fun being but one of them, but it holds no exclusivity. Sometimes, we have to do things that may not be fun at the moment, yet we need to persevere in order to be rewarded later. It's called delayed gratification—be patient.

9. "I'm too busy."

Presidents Reagan, Bush, and Obama, to name but three, all exercised regularly. Are you busier than the POTUS?

10. "My husband/wife gets angry and makes me feel guilty when I leave him/her alone in bed to go to the gym early."

If this is the case, you have more problems than just missing workouts. First, no one has the power to make you feel anything other than you. Second, you're being manipulated by a selfish enabler. Third, you're allowing this to happen. If you fall for this sort of psychological mind game, you will have earned whatever comes next. Go to the gym. Further, if health, fitness, and nutrition are important to you but not to your significant other, file for divorce and do so before you have children. Kids will not improve things because you'll only disagree, bicker, and argue about how best to raise them in a healthful way. Chances are your relationship, such as it is, is spiraling downward at an ever increasing velocity anyway.

11. "Healthy food tastes bad."

False. As a result of bludgeoning our taste buds with the standard American diet (SAD), most Americans taste only three things: sugar, salt and fat. We've basically overwhelmed and wounded our sense of taste. Once you discard the SAD and have experienced approximately two or three months of healthful, nutritious eating, allowing your palate to recover, you will actually taste the food itself for the first time. It's wonderful.

12. "Healthy food isn't real. I want real food."

Healthful food is the very definition of real food. Do you think Lunchables are real food? How about nice, white, squishy Wonder Bread, Twinkies, Sugar Frosted Flakes, Oreos, Pepsi Cola, Coca Cola, Skippy Natural Creamy Peanut Butter with 1/3 less Sodium & Sugar, Reese's Pieces, Doritos? Do you think these qualify as real food? If so, you are terribly mistaken. These items may elicit warm and fuzzy childhood reminiscences due to their being part of your upbringing, but don't confuse the two issues. The only thing real about these harmful creations is that they're "real" bad.

13. "When I go out to dinner with friends, if I order something healthy, they always make fun and question why I eat this way. It's easier to order what they do."

If you can sit there and not preach to them about their abysmal food choices, unless, of course, they ask your advice, they should be able to behave just as politely by refraining from inopportune commentary concerning your food selections. If this seems to be a recurring issue, then they may not be friends worth the trouble of having.

14. "I'm too old to start exercising. It's too late."

As the saying goes, "It's never too late." I recall reading articles where feeble elder folks in their 70s, 80s, and even as old as 90 began consistent, supervised weight training, and in a few months, upon being reevaluated, it was found that they had added lean muscle mass to their frames and had become stronger. You'd be better off starting at a young age, but you can still improve. Exercise works.

15. "I don't need to work out because I have a physically demanding job."

It doesn't matter whether you work heavy construction, landscape, bale hay or chop down trees for a living. Your body adapts to its day-to-day activities. Everyone, regardless of how they're employed, can benefit from a consistent exercise routine. I've known quite a few people who worked at physically demanding jobs and went to the gym right after work.

16. "Regular exercise is boring. I get my exercise by gardening."

Gardening? I like flowers, vegetables, and herbs too, but gardening as an exercise? Gardening is one of the excuses I enjoy hearing the most because it's so ridiculously funny. A variety of other excuses have also been used in its place. Weekend and occasional pastimes which include golfing, tennis, hiking, bowling, squash, table tennis, handball, badminton, basketball, softball, pickleball, paddle ball, canoeing, kayaking, rafting, horseback riding, horseshoe pitching, bocce ball, croquet, darts, ballroom dancing and "chicken-cising" (according to a recent NPR health segment, this is the exercise you get when tending to a flock of flightless birds—I'm not kidding) are all examples of other activities which people have informed me are their exercise choices.

One could argue the technical merits of the above activities being exercise. They are physical in nature and do burn calories. We also burn calories while we sleep. I suppose it depends on what your goals are. From my perspective, the goal that matters most is that of attaining the highest level of health and fitness possible, given certain predetermining factors. The activities delineated above are all enjoyable, but none of them, especially if undertaken when the mood strikes, haphazardly or on the weekends, are going to serve as the cornerstone of a sound fitness regimen. There is no denying that many of these undertakings are physically demanding and difficult to master. While all of these pursuits surely require a certain skill set on the part of the participant, they should be viewed only as supplemental physical activities to a consistent, regimented, daily routine fundamentally rooted in strength training, cardio-pulmonary training, flexibility training and balance training. Participate in any of them if you desire, but do so after your regularly scheduled workout.

I don't believe it's a stretch to say that most serious and professional athletes exert themselves as much during their gym workouts as they do during competition on the field, hardwood, ice, court, apparatus, floor, mat, track, course, in the water and in the ring. Maybe more. Regular workouts that focus on improving the strength, endurance, flexibility, power, speed, balance and quickness of athletes enhance their ability to perform better in their respective sports. It should be noted that these people are performing at the highest levels humanly possible, not hacking about haphazardly or when they have leisure time.

I've also been informed on numerous occasions that vacuuming, dusting, doing laundry and other assorted household chores qualify as exercise. As far as housework is concerned, I would say that most of the country participates in this activity with some semblance of regularity. Most of the country is unfit to a large degree. Obviously, housework isn't getting it done as far as exercise goes.

17. "I have to eat whatever my wife/husband cooks."

You and your significant other need to have a serious heart-to-heart conversation or you need to learn how to cook, or you need to refer back to the last line of excuse number 10 and consider the solution I suggested.

18. "My kids won't eat health food."

I can see who's in charge of this household. You need to reflect upon what kind of example you've set for your children. Let's begin by educating. Referring to real, nutritious food as health food, which is so often used as a derogatory description of food, needs to stop. Teach the children all the benefits of eating real food. Teach them that food that does not maintain or enhance human well-being but, in fact, detracts from health is nothing more than junk food, garbage which pollutes and sickens the body. Learn with your kids about foods that you may have never tried. Slowly introduce these to your family. Let them help you in the preparation of these new foods. Try new cooking techniques. Catering to whiny kids may appear to be the best immediate solution, but in the long term, you will do a great disservice to your loved ones while placing their health and probably their lives at needless risk.

19. "I'm thin, so I don't need to work out, and I can eat whatever I want."

This is absolutely untrue, yet so many thin people fall back on this reasoning. Obviously, the biggest problem with unfit and unhealthy America is the issue of overweight/obesity. The unfit, overweight individuals far outnumber the unfit, thin individuals. But if you're thin, don't be lulled into a false sense of security, which could prove fatal. Thinness doesn't necessarily translate to healthiness or fitness. Plenty of thin people have hypertension, elevated cholesterol, heart disease, cancer, diabetes and suffer strokes. A good number of them can't do more than a handful of pushups, while pull-ups are usually out of the question. The same goes for running as little as one mile. Adequate flexibility is ordinarily non-existent.

Clothing may help the unfit thin disguise their poorly developed bodies, but concealment won't alter the fact that most of these people are concurrently thin and fat or skinny-fat, as this state is sometimes referred to. This condition is typically manifested by presenting a thin appearance, a bodyweight in accordance with actuarial charts but a high percentage of body-fat along with a low percentage of lean muscle mass. I've often heard people proudly declare that they have been the same weight since high school. This commonly means very little, taking into account that the high school weight was undoubtedly the result of a higher percentage of muscle and a lower percentage of fat, while presently, the exact opposite is true. This is why counting calories and being a slave to the scale doesn't work when you strive to become as physically fit and healthy as possible. There's more to this process than simply your weight and becoming thin.

Being physically fit and healthy means developing your body to its peak in whichever stage of life you happen to find yourself, given your specific genetic potential. It doesn't mean fat, skinny, or unnaturally engorged by performance enhancing drugs. The goal is to naturally achieve the highest ratio of lean muscle mass possible as compared to a lower proportion of body-fat through proper nutrition and consistent, challenging exercise. The basic objective for the rational among us should be health, not the endorsement of skinny culture. I'm not advising overweight people to become skinny. I'm suggesting that most of America, regardless of being overweight or thin, is unfit and unhealthy. You can only do the best you can with the means given to you by nature. We can all do better. Change your body composition to one that will optimize your survival and well-being.

20. "I don't need to exercise because I'm very active."

Please refer to the comments under excuse number 15.

21. "I don't eat that way all the time."

This one is hands down, the most frequently repeated and popular of all excuses for consuming poor quality food. I had a gym buddy who was an intelligent, well-educated, and successful man. Every so often, he felt the need to unburden himself from the guilt he was carrying by confessing to me his most recent nutritional sin. Initially, I had attempted to use reason and logic to help him understand the error of his ways. But after repeated transgressions, my patience had evaporated along with any dispensation I might have offered. Perhaps he was a masochist owing to the fact that, by this point, I could extend nothing more than severe lambastings.

One day, during one of our spirited, post-workout, locker room discussions, he felt compelled to inform me that he had eaten a bunch of junk food cookies the night before. He quickly added that he didn't do that all the time. He advised me that later in the day, he was going to a business dinner in New York or Washington, D.C., I don't recall which, but I distinctly remember him saying that he was going to eat scallops wrapped in bacon and drink plenty of vodka. Again, he immediately provided that he didn't eat that way all the time. Just about every time he and I would take part in one of our locker room discourses, the topic would inevitably turn to food and exercise with a heavy emphasis on the food aspect. It seemed to me that he was always eating something that he hardly ever ate except on special occasions or when he was treating himself.

What he refused to see was that he wasn't eating that way (consuming a specific food or beverage) all the time, but he was, in fact, consuming something unhealthful almost all the time. For an individual with this syndrome, and they are legion, the story goes something like this: On Monday night, he eats half a carton of ice cream while watching TV, but he doesn't eat ice cream all the time, so it's okay. On Tuesday night, he eats a bag of potato chips and drinks a liter of Mountain Dew while watching TV. Nonetheless, he doesn't eat potato chips except once in a while and hardly ever drinks soda. On Wednesday, he goes to a late business lunch with a colleague and a client. Lunch lasts a couple of hours, during which time he drinks at least three glasses of wine, eats fettuccine Alfredo (made the REAL food way with white pasta, butter, parmesan cheese and heavy cream), liberally slathers butter on two or three dinner rolls (the REAL kind made with useless white flour), has a couple of after lunch sambucas which are followed by a cup of espresso and a generous chunk of tiramisu. This business lunch has been a success; as such, celebratory cigars are passed around as they exit the restaurant. Not to worry, business luncheons only happen about once every couple of weeks or so. He certainly doesn't eat like this all the time. On Thursday night there's a National Hockey League (NHL) playoff game being aired. He enjoys hockey. He turns on the TV and settles himself comfortably on his couch. During the course of the game, he drinks a few beers, eats oily, salted mixed nuts in addition to Doritos with melted cheddar cheese dip. Hey, he doesn't eat this way all the time. It's the NHL playoffs—they only happen once per year.

Finally, Friday night, the weekend! After a long, tough week at work, everyone looks forward to fun on the weekend. We wish life away to get to the weekend. Alas, one day, we'll all be begging and praying for just one more Monday. All the same, no point thinking about depressing things like that because, as it stands right now, our delusional friend has worked hard the entire week and now it's time to treat himself. The weekend, after all, comes only once a week. It's not like it's the weekend every day.

He, along with his wife, who has also had a demanding week, arrive home at about the same time. After mutually commiserating, they decide that cooking after such a long and laborious week is out of the question. The kids agree as they tune in to HBO, plant themselves on the couch, and order two sausage and pepperoni pizzas with extra cheese and a couple of giant bottles of Diet Coke. Of course they drink Diet Coke as a nod to being conscientious about health. Our friend assuredly doesn't eat pizza all the time, but it's the weekend, and he's sharing quality time with the family.

Saturday breakfasts are always a special treat because his wife has time to cook his favorite: chocolate chip buttermilk pancakes, dripping with real melted butter, and swimming in Log Cabin Syrup (Lite, of course because he's careful about his weight and health). This Saturday morning feast also includes crispy fried bacon—they say everything's better with bacon—spicy sausage patties and American cheese and cream cheese-stuffed omelets. He's mindful to drink a big glass of orange juice to make sure he's receiving his daily quota of vitamin C. He drinks at least two cups of coffee lightened with a non-dairy creamer because, after all, he is watching his calories. As another concession to his health regimen, he only uses two teaspoons of sugar in each cup of coffee instead of the three he used in times prior to his enlightenment concerning wellness. Even though he splurges a little at week's end, no need to go overboard. Moderation is key here, we're talking about his health.

The weatherman smiles on the family Saturday afternoon, so the planned barbecue is on. During this beautiful, sunny day, he drinks frozen margaritas and beer. He eats hot dogs, hamburgers, corn on the cob saturated with salt and butter, potato chips and salted pretzels, salted corn chips, onion dip. German potato salad with "real mayonnaise" is also on the menu. Of course it's made with "real mayonnaise," or what's the point? It's the weekend and he plows ahead with deviled eggs, baked pork and beans and finally, ice cream cake. What a great All-American time. Fun on the weekend! How normal to have family and friends around enjoying one another as they stuff themselves with heart stopping food and drink akin to a Roman orgy. Culture, tradition, fun, real food and drink, family, friends, "all normal," God Bless America!

Sunday morning, everyone sleeps in after having partied late into the night. Nevertheless, they make sure to attend church, being a God-fearing family. After services, it's time to take advantage of the last day of the weekend and treat the family to brunch at a local hotel renowned for these feasts. Tomorrow it will be back to the grind, so he deserves a bit of an indulgence. He drinks mimosas and fancy coffees laden with whipped cream and chocolate. He eats a small cheese omelet to leave room for the eggs Benedict with real hollandaise sauce. He engluts a moderate-sized strip steak and partakes of a slice of Taylor ham along with an order of home fries. The cheese-stuffed crepes topped with sweetened fruit are a delight. The flaky white buttered and jellied biscuits, sugar-glazed buns and warm, buttery apple turnovers encrusted with more sweet, sugary glaze beckon and he is quick to acquiesce.

It's a good thing he doesn't do this all the time or he would gain more weight than he's already gained. The way he looks at it, with all the hard work he puts in at the gym, when time allows of course, he deserves to treat himself—to live, as he so often puts it. Although, he's perplexed as to why the workouts aren't paying off. He's fatter than ever and getting fatter. Maybe a new gym, a new workout routine, or a new trainer will do the trick.

Dinner at home this Sunday evening consists of Saturday's barbecue leftovers. It's amazing that anyone can cram another morsel of food into themselves after that terrific brunch but that was hours ago, and everyone's hungry now. The family heats up the leftovers, piles the plates high, and gathers around the TV to enjoy the latest Netflix presentation, wringing out every bit of living the weekend has to offer.

Does anyone detect a predicament here? Do you notice a troubling pattern? Our friend has himself convinced that he's overseeing his health. He's managed this feat by refusing to look at his overall behaviors, ergo, failing to take responsibility for those behaviors. This is made possible by simply compartmentalizing his abysmal dietary habits. To say that he doesn't eat that way all the time is technically correct. In his mind, each poor food choice stands alone.

Each calendar year consists of 365 days, except for the leap year. Each year embodies 52 weeks. If you accept Friday as the beginning of the weekend, it follows that there are 3 weekend days every week. A little simple math (52 x 3 = 156) illustrates that there are 156 days to treat yourself because it's the weekend. Bear in mind that we're only calling attention to weekend treats at this point.

When we analyze the overall picture, what we expose is a cycle of insanity. Besides weekends, we all know that there are other "infrequent" days when we treat ourselves because it's a special occasion. Let's take a look at these additional days starting with New Year's Day. Last night's party has come and gone. The common thinking is that it's time for a fresh start, to hit the gym, go on a diet and get into shape. Before you know it, summer will arrive and you have to look good.

You make it through January mostly unscathed, except of course, for the weekend indulgences. Now it's February and time for a Super Bowl party, which must include chips, dips, booze, hoagies, meat lovers pizzas (because everyone knows that real men watch football and eat meat), and much, much more. Even though February is the shortest month, it's a great one. You really get bang for the buck as a result of Valentine's Day adding to the gastronomical ecstasies experienced on weekends and the Super Bowl blowout. Ah, Valentine's Day, with chocolates, sweets, romantic, candle-lit restaurant dinners with your beloved and whatever else you eat and drink in the name of love.

March ushers in St. Patrick's Day soaked in alcohol to go along with that culinary delight, corned beef. Add to this the numerous social gatherings replete with the type of food and drink associated with watching sports, specifically centered around the increasingly popular National Collegiate Athletic Association (NCAA) Men's and Women's Division 1 Basketball Tournaments, commonly referred to as March Madness. These tournaments last about three weeks. We can see that this month provides much needed, ample respites from the daily drudgeries of life by offering that rare opportunity to treat ourselves with food and drink. March Madness, indeed. It should be noted that the January resolution to begin a consistent workout program carried through to early March where it waned and ultimately died. Why? Scan the list of excuses and insert the one you like best.

Late March or early April, depending on where the days fall on the calendar, brings us Palm Sunday and Easter dinners in all their glory. But they don't really count because they both occur on a weekend day and that would be unfair. Still and all, the children are gorging on chocolate Easter bunnies, jelly beans, cream-filled chocolate eggs and gnawing the heads off of marshmallow peeps. In the blink of an eye, it's May, which heralds the much anticipated season of summer here in the northern hemisphere. It kicks off with Memorial Day and its associated weekend. Cookouts and beach food rule this time of year. July in the United States of America brings with it Independence Day. Another day of barbecues, beer and general feasting culminating in a fireworks extravaganza. What's not to like? Summer treats continue through August because it's, well, summer.

With September comes Labor Day weekend, the last hurrah and unofficial end of summer. What better way to bid this season adieu than with another massive barbecue? October, and can you believe it's Halloween already? Time flies when you're eating your way through the year. Not only are your kids stuffing themselves with handfuls of candy, you've been caught in the act of stealing it from them again.

With November comes Thanksgiving. Thanksgiving Day to New Year's Day is a five to six-week spectacle of eating and drinking ourselves into a coma at a seemingly endless number of holiday parties. Time to celebrate! That's why it's called the holiday season, that wondrous time of year beginning with Thanksgiving and including Hanukkah, Christmas, Kwanzaa, and New Year's Eve. This isn't simply a day or a weekend but an entire season devoted to gorging and gluttony. What's the excuse this time? "It's the holidays. I don't eat that way all the time."

As if this weren't enough when you add to the previous tally the occasional birthday, baptism, communion, confirmation, bar mitzvah, bat mitzvah, wedding, graduation, promotion, retirement, engagement, bachelor and bachelorette party, funeral, family reunion, company picnic, vacation, social visit, sporting event attendance, welcome home, going away, block party, feast, carnival, county fair, circus, zoo visit, movie theater excursion and so many more instances where eating and drinking are integrated into and on par with the main event, you're left with one hell of a lot of days that are special occasions. But there's more. Take the weekends and special occasions and add to them all the celebrations particular to each race, region, ethnicity, and religion that I haven't even touched upon. Finally, include those regular days during the week in which you're pigging out on a different disease promoting food almost continuously.

I don't think it's a stretch to say that there are about 230 days during the year that are special occasions and treat-yourself days, and I'm probably being generous with my count. That's 230 out of 365 days or 63% of the time spent treating yourself. You're treating yourself more than half the time. Eating "that way" is exactly what you do most of the time. It's your chosen way of life. In fact, the special occasion seems to be when you're not eating in a manner consistent with killing yourself.

This revolving food orgy is further exacerbated by either no exercise on your part or misguided and spiritless attempts at exercise. There is no way in which golf or gardening could possibly counteract the caloric and toxic avalanche thundering down your gaping maw and into your ever-expanding gut. Unless your idea of gardening is cutting down half of the Amazonian rainforest with a hatchet or you're sprinting between holes on the golf course carrying both your golf bag and golf cart on your back every day, you're extremely likely to gain unhealthful weight and/or damage your body in ways that are not immediately observable. Know that excuses are not good reasons to do or not do something. They are nothing more than an avoidance of reality. Your health and peace of mind will be much better served if you're honest with yourself.

It's not beyond the realm of rational thought that all mentally stable individuals desire good health. The question is, what are they willing to contribute toward this goal? You can pray for good health and hope for the best, which sounds like playing the lottery to me. You can also wrangle some control away from the fates by doing your part. However, you won't start doing what you need to until your desire for good health overtakes your desire for harmful food, drink and habits. To be your best, you must radically change your thinking. Anything short of this, resorting to buzzwords like moderation and treats and the implementation of excuses will result in failure. When you are ready to stand alone, when need be, only then will you abandon excuses and embark on a crusade for your best health.

When you experience this reality check, you admit to yourself that you have been your own worst enemy. You acknowledge that you are ready for meaningful and significant change. You set a well-thought-out, intelligent and logical plan into motion by making a decision to educate yourself about nutrition, exercise, and health in general. As you experience this epiphany of sorts, you'll realize that fad diets don't work, hucksters on TV at 2:00 AM selling ab machines and magic pills won't help your weight problem and that you're ready, finally, to commit to a lifestyle change, no matter what.

When the positive changes to your overall health and appearance become perceptible, you will experience the greatest treat of all. The trip to your doctor's office for your annual physical will become an opportunity for you to gloat as a result of the great numbers presented in your blood work. The doctor will notice that your resting heart rate and blood pressure have gone down. Additionally, unless your illnesses legitimately result from something other than your previously lousy lifestyle, your doctor will be able to lessen, if not, discontinue the various medications you needed when you were full of excuses.

What an indulgence it will be to step out of the shower, look in the mirror and know that you are the best that you can be. It certainly beats cringing when you look at yourself. This is a success. The aim is to physically and mentally be able to enjoy life for as long as possible, not to sabotage a beautiful gift with lame excuses.

18

Standing Alone

Whatever happened to the fierce, independent spirit of Americans? To a certain degree a number of us remain individualistic, but some behaviors persist in which most of us are predictably alike, usually to our individual detriment. The best example of this like-minded thinking can be easily detected by studying our practices concerning health, fitness and nutrition.

Most humans celebrate holidays and special occasions with copious amounts of bad food and drink. Commonly, people can't wait for the weekend to arrive, hence, TGIF. The majority eats a variety of harm-inducing food during the work week, making a bad joke out of statements such as, "I can't wait for the weekend, so I can eat what I want." The implication is that they are living a nutritionally monastic life. Apart from historical times of need and want, nearly all Americans have always been eating exactly what they desire and continue to do so with no realistic end in sight. The preponderance of the population is picnicking, partying, barbecuing and holds that there's absolutely nothing wrong with foods and beverages such as, but certainly not limited to, hamburgers, hot dogs, beer, apple pie, ice cream, soda, potato chips, wine, donuts, coffee, pizza, candy, cake, fat steaks, fast food in general and deep-fried anything. Given a choice, most choose unwisely. That's easy enough to see by simply looking around.

Thoughtless eating and its resulting medical problems are magnified by the fact that meaningful exercise is an activity that is overwhelmingly loathed and avoided. This is an indisputable recipe for a dreadful health outcome. As a result of our suicidal nutritional and exercise tendencies, at the very least, our health suffers. It follows that medical intervention becomes necessary. Doctors provide pills and assorted drugs, which have their own potential for endangering patient health due to the possibility of adverse side effects. If the medications don't restore us to eating shape, then medically invasive procedures are always a consideration. Arriving at this point, you become part of the disease management system. Your life revolves around visits to the doctor and the pharmacy interspersed with frustrating, time-consuming, emotionally draining and life-sucking phone calls to your health insurance provider. The vast majority of the time, and I can't emphasize this enough, your infirmity is self-inflicted. This is what passes for normal in America. This is the system and way of life the majority considers acceptable.

If we're fortunate enough at birth, and most are, we are given a gift, a perfectly running machine and at a later date it's as if we say to ourselves, "This seems to be running nicely; how can I fuck it up?" It's the equivalent of receiving a brand new Bentley and never tuning it up, never changing the oil, never doing any of the required maintenance and as a result, running it into the ground. One day, you jump in and lo and behold, it doesn't start. You sit there and actually wonder why.

Those of us who have rejected the cultural norms surrounding eating and drinking, not to mention the plethora of other senseless activities embraced by the normal majority, have quietly staged individual revolutions. We are radical in our beliefs and practices, which is so very sad because there is nothing radical about our goal—optimal health. This shouldn't even be an issue because it's so basic. We have rejected a mind-numbing culture that promotes behaviors that lead to grotesque body proportions, sickness and ultimate self-destruction. We realize the importance of preventative maintenance. We want to be like the classic muscle cars from the 1960s and 1970s, still running well and looking good today, years after they've left Detroit.

Regrettably, we are the smallest of minorities. Fanatics, eccentrics, neurotics, food police, narcissists, food Nazis, gym rats and health nuts are but some of the mocking labels attributed to those of our ilk. We are seen as frustrated, miserable, uptight, unhappy, intense type-A personalities who wouldn't know a good time if it bit us in our collectively tight, muscular asses. We mostly stand alone. This takes tremendous will and an unyielding strength of conviction. I, for one, wouldn't have it any other way. Standing alone in this instance, means being a critical thinker. When it comes to eating and drinking, it's generally a good idea that when you see the crowd running in a particular direction, run for your life in the opposite direction. People do many stupid things. Why should it be any different with their health?

Isn't it ironic that those who treasure and work at improving and preserving their health are called health nuts? How should we refer to those people who abuse and ultimately destroy their health? Are they the sanely unhealthy? When the time comes, don't be afraid to stand alone if necessary. Be a proud health nut. They say we are extreme. I'll repeat what extreme is for those of you who may have glossed over my initial description of extreme, in Chapter 17. That's when the surgeon, in a desperate, life-saving attempt, splits your sternum like a chicken in order to reveal your chest cavity, granting him access to what's left of the heart you have destroyed by treating yourself with all that fun food. Having a festering wound that refuses to heal on an appendage or limb due to complications from diabetes, resulting in that body part being cleaved—now, we're talking extreme. Standing alone doesn't look like such a bad idea when you examine the issues from a realistic, unvarnished perspective. Be prudent, be strong, reject the preposterous behaviors, and stand alone. Your life depends on it.

19

White Flour

The primary component of nearly all the breads, cakes, cookies, muffins, and sundry baked goods available at grocery stores and other locations is white flour, usually referred to on packaging as enriched wheat flour. To the nutritionally apathetic, the use of the adjective *enriched*, engenders a positive feeling. Why would it not? How can something described as enriched have a negative connotation? As beneficial as enriched wheat flour may appear, it is nothing more than white flour. That is precisely where the shoe pinches because the negative aspects of consuming white flour far outweigh the positives of the enrichment process.

When a whole grain, in this case wheat, is processed and converted into white flour, nearly all the vitamins, minerals and fiber are ground out of the whole grain. What remains is a virtually worthless, simple carbohydrate, almost pure starch. Living organisms, humans included, require proper food from which they can extract the vast array of nutrients—vitamins, minerals, fiber etc., essential for life. This is why people are *supposed* to eat. For the purpose of returning some nutrimental value to this degraded white powder, the processors *enrich*, or add back some of the vitamins and minerals they removed in the initial conversion process. They reintegrate to the white flour what the scientific community deems important based on current knowledge.

The more scientists study food and nutrition, the more they realize and readily admit that they don't know about this subject. As I brought to your attention earlier when elaborating on science, they fail to accept the complex relationships among all of a food's integrants. They ignore how both known and yet to be discovered components of food interact and may interact with one another in providing health benefits to the consumer. What they add back to the flour is based on conventional wisdom. Could scientists be failing to include some very important nutrients during the enrichment process? This is almost certain. Is the food more healthful when enriched rather than if it had remained as a whole grain? Positively not. Then why is enriching practiced?

Whole grains are mainly composed of three elements, the bran, which is the outer portion of the grain, the germ which is the seed's embryo and the endosperm which serves as the source of nutrients for the growing embryo. The bran contains mostly insoluble fiber, some minerals and a bit of protein. The germ includes B vitamins, some minerals and fat. The endosperm is made up of carbohydrates, soluble fiber, protein, some B vitamins and iron.

In times before modern technology it wasn't possible to grind cereal grains down to the powdery consistency achievable today. Old time bread was gritty and dense but didn't last long before it would get moldy and otherwise decay. The reason for the short shelf life was that during the primitive grinding process, the germ was crushed, releasing the fat, which when exposed to the air would begin to putrefy. With the implementation of more efficient methods of grinding, it became possible to separate the carbohydrate rich endosperm from the rest of the grain. Once the problematic, fatty oil-containing germ was removed from the equation, the result was a fine powdery flour that remained hardy for an extended period of time. Only those who could afford to eat refined-flour white bread did so. As such, it became a matter of elevating one's social status to eat white bread made from this refined flour. The term peasant bread exists for a reason. The poor couldn't afford white bread and continued to subsist on unrefined, whole grain, gritty, crusty bread.

What the early producers and consumers of refined grains failed to realize was that there was a downside to manufacturing a bread that would retain freshness for a longer period of time, was easier to digest and provided social status. The down side was that once the bran and germ were removed from the whole grain, the result was a product significantly reduced in nutrients and culpable in the initiation of preventable disease. What remained was mostly a simple starch, in other words, sugar. This sugar could be quickly absorbed by the blood. In simple terms, when a high sugar content food is consumed, the body responds by tasking the pancreas to produce insulin to lower blood sugar to acceptable levels. It's well known that repeated consumption of easily and quickly digestible sugary foods can unduly tax the pancreas, potentially leading to obesity, type II diabetes and heart disease.

Years later, it was discovered that refining grains substantially degraded their nutritional value. However, by this point refined-grain white bread was commonly accepted in most areas. In an effort to improve the nutritional quality of the bread, the process of enriching white flour was introduced.

As you can see, white flour was not advocated for its health promoting appeal. I suppose a pro-health argument could be made that eating moldy bread had the potential to sicken people. But human nature being what it is, extended shelf life (better for sales) and appearance of the product were more than likely a greater influence for the use of white flour than the general wellness of the population. Furthermore, people were unaware of insulin spikes in blood sugar, let alone its causes, and ignorant about the importance of dietary fiber. This lack of knowledge concurrent with the thinking of the day, to produce a bread that was quickly and easily digested was no cause for concern. Instead, it was celebrated.

The core of the issue is that no matter the genesis of white bread and its subsequent evolution into modern, enriched-flour white bread, it remains a poor substitute for whole grain flour, as do all processed grains. By using the terms *enriched* and *wheat flour* on the packaging of goods containing grains, unsuspecting consumers are duped into believing that they are purchasing a healthful product. The use of these words is, plainly, a brilliant marketing ploy on the part of food producers. A confused, ignorant and gullible consumer is a food producer's dream come true. They are ready, willing and quite able to exploit the naive public. They're counting on your lack of knowledge and literally banking on your faith and trust in them, along with their allies in government and advertising. Manufacturers of inferior foods masquerading as wholesome foods rule the market. Grocery stores are repositories for mostly poor food.

To their own detriment, many consumers play right into the hands of food producers who push white enriched flour and other processed grains. I've frequently heard people say that they don't like whole grains, especially when speaking about bread and pasta. Their reasons range from describing whole grains as *too chewy* to *too gritty*. Some have said they don't care for the appearance of whole grain breads and pastas, adding that they don't taste like the *real* thing. It makes no difference if what they're used to eating is no more than a substandard bastardization of wholesome food, to them it's real. Getting people to think this way is an example of marketing at its best. The truth is that 100% whole grain is the real food, while enriched white flour is basically a nutritional abomination that plays a significant role in disease promotion.

Whole grains require more work for the body to digest. This is a positive outcome when they are eaten. They require more time to pass through the digestive tract because they are tougher to break down due to their high fiber content. They release their sugars at a much slower rate than quickly digested refined-flour products. This causes a less dramatic blood glucose spike and subsequent insulin response from your already overworked pancreas. Whole grains keep you fuller longer, increasing the time between meals. When you eat refined grains or foods made with them, they are quickly absorbed and turned into glucose. This is problematic because soon you're hungry and ready to eat again. Perhaps you've heard of the old allegation that people are hungry an hour after eating Chinese food. What they're probably referring to is the American interpretation of Chinese food, which is low in protein and fiber. White rice is the equivalent of white flour, devoid of most of its original nutrients, including all of its fiber. Again, it's basically a useless starch quickly converted by the body into glucose. Of course, you're going to be hungry soon after such a meal.

When purchasing any packaged food, in this specific case, foods that start out as whole grains, like flour, baked goods and cereals, pay close attention to the information on the label. Sometimes a little information is a bad thing. You can be easily fooled into buying something that you thought was healthful when the reality is just the opposite. Beware of labels such as "Contains Real Whole Grains," "Whole Grain Blend," or "Contains Wheat" and similar claims. It's of paramount importance that you realize and remember that you are your best health and wellness advocate. Never forget that food producers and marketers are masters at what they do. They want you to purchase their products and will do whatever it takes to entice you to do so. They are virtuosos in the art of deception, manipulation, propaganda and lying, usually without actually lying.

A product labeled "Made With Real Whole Grains" may in fact contain real whole grains. Not much of any item needs to be included in a particular food for that product to lay claim to the fact that it contains that item. This holds true even if the real whole grains added amounted to only 5% of the total product. By way of illustration, a loaf of bread can be 95% enriched wheat flour (white flour) and 5% whole wheat flour and announce, "Made With Real Whole Grains." Technically, this isn't a lie. The reality, however, is that the bread is almost entirely made of white flour. The sellers count on you, the consumer, armed with just enough knowledge, to spot the assertion "Whole Grains" on the package and respond in knee-jerk fashion. Most shoppers are in a hurry, distracted and thinking about other things to feel the need to investigate further upon seeing "Whole Grains" on a label. They've learned just enough to know that whole grains are the far superior choice, and into the shopping cart goes a loaf of bread that is 95% white flour.

Some breads and other products may contain greater proportions of whole grains than white flour. This remains unacceptable when 100% whole grain products are available. If you're working to be your best, your food choices need to be the best you can find. Keep your food standards high by not permitting any amount of an ingredient that you know to be inferior into your food. Move away from the wishy-washy attitude of moderation when it comes to ingesting any food that you recognize doesn't measure up. Stand firm, and don't compromise your health or that of your family. Eat 100% whole grains. White flour should be banished from people's diets and unceremoniously relegated to art classes for making papier-mâché. That's one purpose for which it's well suited.

20

High Fructose Corn Syrup

Corn syrup is corn sugar or dextrose. It's a sweet syrup made from cornstarch by the chemical process known as hydrolysis. High fructose corn syrup (HFCS) is a group of corn syrups that has been processed, changing its glucose to fructose. It's then mixed with pure corn syrup, which is 100% glucose. This process produces the intended sweetness. The variations of HFCS available on the market are dependent upon what percentage of it is combined with fructose and glucose. All have different applications with different food products.

In the United States, HFCS is found in nearly all processed food and drink. Besides being generally found in institutional food, including school food, HFCS is, more specifically speaking, part of many ice creams, baking mixes, cookies, salad dressings, soups, peanut butters, breads, candies, sherbets, cakes, hams, bacons, sausages, ketchups, luncheon meats, cheeses, canned vegetables, carbonated beverages, Chinese foods, alcoholic beverages, and numerous other foods and drinks. As you can see, the list is varied and extensive.

HFCS is used as a sugar replacement because it's easier to mix with other ingredients and convey from one location to another due to its liquid form. Also, HFCS is a little cheaper in America than sugar due to laws implemented in the mid-1970s which increased the cost of sugar imports. The price of corn is cheap in the U.S. as a result of subsidies paid by the federal government to the farmers who grow it. This prompts farmers to produce more and more corn every year and glut the marketplace with it.

It's worth noting that since about the mid-1970s when HFCS began its infiltration of practically all processed foods, a correlation was discovered between rising obesity rates in America over the last three or four decades or so and the increased consumption of HFCS. The relatively low cost of HFCS and its ubiquity in nearly all processed foods and soft drinks has led to a far greater consumption of sugars by the populace. In fact, HFCS, ironically enough, is easily found in many so-called health or meal replacement bars widely available in health food stores.

An individual may decide to take control of his life and health by eliminating obvious sugar-laden culprits such as snack cakes, cookies, candy and soda. But if he's not aware of the various forms of sugars quietly hiding in the processed foods he continues to consume, his health will remain at high risk. These sugars contribute what are known as empty calories to our diet. This means that these foods contain more energy than most whole foods, especially when the sugars in these processed foods are combined with fats. They contain more energy in the form of calories, not in actual nutrients. To the uninitiated, hearing or reading that a particular food contains more energy than another food appears to be an endorsement of the higher energy food. You have to pay attention because this is absolutely untrue. These high energy concoctions made up of sugar, fat, and salt are virtually devoid of fiber and important micronutrients (vitamins and minerals). The ones that do contain even smidgeons of useful nutrients remain poor choices because of their combination with undesirable ingredients. If your objective is health, you'd do well to stay away from HFCS and corn syrup.

21

Hydrogenated Oil

Hydrogenation is the process whereby oils which are liquid at room temperature, are converted into semisolid fats at room temperature. This is accomplished by introducing hydrogen gas under high pressure to those liquid oils. Examples are margarine, shortening and Crisco. Usually, the more a fat becomes hydrogenated, the more the fat becomes saturated. This is bad news for anyone eating foods containing these oils. On the other hand, it works well for processed food manufacturers because the shelf life of their products is increased by adding hydrogenated oils to these sickening creations. The increase in shelf life is affected owing to the fact that hydrogenation makes it much more difficult for food to spoil or for the degeneration of its flavor due to oxidation. Both vegetable and animal fats can be hydrogenated. The more solid an oil becomes, the more hydrogenated it is. Hydrogenated oils have a higher melting point. As a result, they are used in deep frying.

It's interesting to note that when partially hydrogenated oil was first introduced, especially in the form of margarine, it was touted as a healthful substitute in place of fatty butter. Commonly accepted is the idea that unsaturated fats are better for health than saturated fats due to their ability, in some cases, to lower the so-called "bad cholesterol," known as low-density lipoproteins (LDL), in our blood. The unstable fatty acids in oils are unsaturated fats. Due to the instability of these fatty acids, they are quicker to become rancid. Unfortunately for the consumer, when oil is hydrogenated, promoting longer shelf life for products, the healthful fats are chemically altered into another type of fatty acid called a trans-fat. The type of trans-fat I'm referring to here is artificial, not the natural trans-fats produced by bacteria found in the guts of ruminants such as cows and sheep.

Years ago, the media discovered and began to heavily report on the health risks of eating foods containing trans-fat. These fats can significantly contribute to the development of coronary heart disease. Trans-fats are potentially deadly because they have the ability to increase LDL and decrease the so-called "good cholesterol," known as high-density lipoproteins (HDL). As bad for your health as saturated fats may be, it seems that trans-fats may be worse. They increase triglycerides which are fats found in your blood and stored in other fat cells to be used as a later source of energy. In this manner, they serve a purpose in certain body functions. However, when blood triglyceride levels become too elevated, they can contribute to heart disease.

Some cities in America actually tried to reduce their citizens' consumption of trans-fats. In 2006, New York City was the first large city in the U.S. to limit its use in restaurants. Other cities and locations in America including Philadelphia, San Francisco and Chicago followed suit and issued partial bans on trans-fats or implemented voluntary programs on the part of restaurants to cease their use. In 2015, the U. S. Food and Drug Administration (FDA) banned the use of trans-fats and gave food makers until 2018 to eliminate them from their products.

While this appears to have been a resounding victory in the name of health, it was only a partial victory. Due to the political nature of banning anything, toxic or not, which shouldn't even be a consideration, compromises and exemptions were made. Manufacturers that produced foods containing trans-fats before the 2018 deadline went into effect were given permission to sell them until January 2020 and in some cases, later. Some food exceptions from the trans-fat ban include varieties of margarine, microwavable popcorn, baked goods, fried fast foods, non-dairy coffee creamers, chips, and a host of other products. It's plain to see that the word *ban* was used in a figurative sense.

In a just and righteous world the health and well-being of the people would always take precedence. Sadly, there exists in our world a great deal that is unjust, which oftentimes overpowers what is just. In America the almighty dollar reigns supreme. A clear illustration of the type of pandering in which our feckless legislators and governmental policymakers engage with powerful food industry interests can be seen in trans-fat labeling. It's perfectly legal for a package of processed food to be labeled as containing 0 grams of trans-fat if the product incorporates less than 0.5 grams of trans-fat per serving. Think about this for a moment. This means that a serving of this "0 trans-fat" food product could potentially be carrying as much as 0.49 grams of trans-fat per serving. If you were a person who had decided to begin living like you cared, this would be a problem. Allowing that you ate only three meals each day with no snacking but were ignorant about this FDA-approved legerdemain, thereby contributing to your consumption of trans-fats at every meal, you could potentially ingest 1.47 grams of trans-fats every day. Based on my unofficial studies, most people probably eat more than three times per day. In addition, particularly in the case of the overweight, how many in this group do you think are eating one serving of anything?

Even the American Heart Association, an institution which I feel is often reserved in its advice, recommends limiting your consumption of trans-fats to less than 2 grams per day, or about 1% of your daily calories, based on a 2,000 calories daily average diet. Conservatively speaking, with only one of these phony 0 trans-fat servings at each of three meals, you could be taking in almost 75% of your recommended daily limit. Remember, this doesn't include additional servings or snacks. For someone eating three servings of fake 0 trans-fat food per day, the math could conceivably look like this: 1.47 grams of trans-fat x 365 days/year = 536.55 grams of trans-fats consumed per year. Further, many fast foods like french fries, deep fried onion rings and chicken nuggets can meet or exceed that 2 grams daily limit of trans-fat in just one serving. Zero trans-fats? No, once again, smoke and mirrors by food companies aided and abetted by our government. A clear case of very creative lying.

Trans-fats pose a grave danger to our health by contributing to coronary heart disease. There are more than enough worthless, disease promoting foods and beverages available for those among us who choose to consume them. We don't need to permit yet another one, especially in light of what is known about the nature of these toxins. As a matter of public health policy, trans-fats should be banned in the literal sense with no more time wasted on studies, committees or discussions. They aren't remotely close to being a necessary nutrient for humans, not even in moderation and instead threaten our well-being. Get rid of them.

22

Salt

Table salt is a refined salt mostly made up of sodium chloride. The sodium chloride content of salt can range from approximately 60% to 99%. After salt is collected it must be purified, which usually involves recrystallization, a process by which chemicals are added to a solution to remove any unwanted material, most often in the form of calcium and magnesium salts. The purified salt is then dried. Anti-caking agents are added once the salt has recrystallized. Potassium iodide is added for iodized salt.

Salt (sodium and chloride) is necessary for humans and other animals to live. It controls the body's fluid balance and plays a role in nerve and muscle function. Too little salt in the diet can cause serious health problems. This however, is not the concern in the United States today. Our issue is an overconsumption of salt. At present, depending on who's disseminating the advice, the generally accepted, maximum, healthful daily allotment for salt in our diet stands at approximately 1,500 mg-2,300 mg or in terms of grams, 1.5 grams-2.3 grams. To translate these numbers into a more familiar format so that you can plainly see how relatively small an amount this is, 2,300 mg of sodium is about equal to the amount of salt held in a teaspoon. You can see by these numbers that a teaspoon or less is all the salt necessary for maintaining vital body functions.

There are many examples of healthful foods which contain naturally occurring sodium, which is one of the most plentiful elements on our planet. Most whole foods contain at least some degree of sodium. Of course, the amount of sodium will vary depending on the soil conditions in which the foods are grown, the mass and measurable amount of the particular food in question and other factors. Most people I've spoken to have been unaware of the fact that sodium occurs naturally in plant-based foods. To give you a general idea of good foods that don't commonly come to mind when thinking about salt, I've listed some of the foods containing naturally occurring sodium. There are many others.

They include:

1-kale (raw, half cup chopped) 15 mg

2-yam (raw, half cup, diced) 7 mg

3-zucchini (fresh with skin, half cup, chopped) 2 mg

4-garbanzo beans (dry, quarter cup) 10 mg

5-lima beans (dry, quarter cup) 20 mg

6-lentils (dry, quarter cup) 15 mg

7-carrot (raw, 1) 40 mg

8-cabbage (raw, shredded, half cup) 6 mg

9-beet (fresh, about 2" in diameter) 64 mg

10-cauliflower (raw, 3.5 ounces) 30 mg

11-broccoli (fresh, 1 medium stalk) 55 mg

12-raisins (quarter cup) 5-10 mg

13-blueberries (fresh, half cup) 5 mg

14-celery (fresh, 2 stalks) 100 mg

15-green onion (raw, quarter cup) 5 mg

16-pistachio nuts (dry roasted, unsalted, 1 ounce) 2 mg

17-spinach (fresh, 3 ounces) 65-160 mg

18-sunflower seeds (dry roasted, unsalted, 10 ounces) 1 mg

When we eat a healthful, whole food, plant-based diet and tally the daily amount of sodium we are eating, we realize that we're getting all the sodium we need from this type of diet. Most of the added, unnecessary and potentially damaging sodium we ingest comes from processed food, fast food and restaurant food. The majority of Americans haven't a clue as to how much overall salt they're consuming and due to the standard American diet (SAD), get nearly double the maximum recommended amount of sodium. Some people are more sensitive than others to the blood pressure raising characteristics of sodium and place themselves at greater risk for potentially life-threatening health problems. Those with hypertension, kidney disease, diabetes, the elderly and African-Americans are particularly susceptible to these risks.

Overconsumption of sodium has been linked to fluid retention (edema), ulcers, heart disease, stroke and as mentioned above and commonly known, hypertension. Over the years, as people have been eating more and more substandard food, which is heavily salted, our taste buds have become inured to salt. As a result, we require more salt to be able to actually taste it. Many people are not only unaware of how much sodium they ingest, but they're also oblivious to the vast variety of food products in which added sodium is hidden, often in stunning amounts.

What are some examples of sodium content in what I consider to be substandard foods? It's very easy to find this information. The next time you visit the grocery store, all you need to do is examine the nutrition label on a food product you're interested in researching. If you don't want to wait for your next food shopping run, simply perform an online search. The information is freely and conveniently accessible. I compiled a random sampling of numerous foods which contain, from a health perspective, unneeded and possibly health damaging, added sodium. Bear in mind that most of the listed foods contain a surplus of other problematic ingredients including fats, sugar, cholesterol, artificial colors, white flour and difficult to pronounce chemicals not fit for the health-minded to consume. In addition and predictably, some packaged products of devalued food were emblazoned with the health claims I pointed out earlier. For our purposes here, I'm simply going to focus on sodium.

At the time of my informal and unofficial research, this was the sodium content of arbitrarily selected substandard foods and meals:

1-Pepperidge Farm, White, Sliced Bread, Original (serving size-2 slices) 210 mg

2-Hormel, Kid's Kitchen, Beans & Wieners (serving size-220 g=1 container) 780 mg

3-Baskin-Robbins Ice Cream, Non-Dairy & Vegan Chocolate Chip Cookie Dough (serving size-1 scoop=2.5 oz.) 80 mg

4-Hunt's Barbeque Sauce, Smoked Flavors, Hickory Cracked Pepper (serving size-36 g=2 tbsp) 160 mg

5-Boar's Head Canadian Style Uncured Bacon (serving size-2 oz.) 480 mg

6-MorningStar Farms Veggie Bacon Strips (serving size-2 strips=16 g) 220 mg

7-Blimpie Blimp Sub (serving size-large) 5,390 mg

8-Blimpie Tuna Sub (serving size-regular) 870 mg

9-Blimpie Meatball Parmigiana Sub (serving size-large) 4,170 mg

10-Blimpie Kid's Subs, Tuna (serving size-3") 510 mg

11-Bob Evans Farm Fresh Egg Combinations (Country-Fried Steak & Farm-Fresh Eggs with Fried Eggs, Sausage, Grits and Specialty Bread) 3,640 mg

12-Bob Evans Breakfast Sausage Classics (Sausage Gravy Breakfast with Home Fries) 3,020 mg

13-Burger King (Bacon & Cheese Whopper) 1,560 mg

14-Burger King (BK Veggie Burger) 980 mg

15-Burger King (Double Quarter Pound King) 1,810 mg

16-Yves Veggie Cuisine Gluten Free Veggie Burger-Plant-based (serving size-1 patty=75 g) 400 mg

17-Yves Veggie Cuisine Veggie Pepperoni-Plant-based (serving size-10 slices=30 g) 260 mg

18-Yves Veggie Cuisine Veggie Turkey-Plant-based (serving size-5 slices=51 g) 300 mg

19-Dr. Praeger's California Veggie Burger (serving size-1 burger=113 g) 310 mg

20-General Mills Wheat Chex Cereal (serving size-0.75 cup) 268 mg

21-Cascadian Farm Raisin Bran Cereal (serving size-1 ¼ cup) 290 mg

22-Malt-O-Meal Toasty O'S Cereal (serving size-1 cup=30 g) 269 mg

23-Post Grape-Nuts Cereal (serving size-1/2 cup=2 oz.) 270 mg

24-Kellogg's Smart Start Strong Heart Maple Brown Sugar Cereal (serving size-1 ¼ cup) 140 mg

25-Kellogg's Rice Krispies Cereal, Original (serving size-1 cup=28 g) 190 mg

26-General Mills Cheerios (serving size-0.75 cup=27 g) 172 mg

27-Kraft Cheez Whiz Medium Salsa Con Queso (serving size-2 tbsp) 500 mg

28-Kraft American Cheese Singles (serving size-1 slice=21 g) 220 mg

29-Alpine Lace Reduced Fat Swiss Cheese (serving size-23 g) 90 mg

30-Panera Bread Broccoli Cheddar Soup (serving size-1 bowl) 1,330 mg

31-Panera Bread Low-Fat Chicken Noodle Soup (serving size-1 bowl) 1,490 mg

32-Panera Bread Ten Vegetable Soup (serving size-1 bowl) 1,090 mg

33-Heinz Simply Heinz Tomato Ketchup (serving size-1 tbsp) 160 mg

34-Kentucky Fried Chicken, Limited Time Offer (Chicken & Donut Sandwich) 1,310 mg

35-Kentucky Fried Chicken (Original Recipe Chicken Breast) 1,190 mg

36-Kentucky Fried Chicken (Honey BBQ Sandwich) 1,350 mg

37-Arby's (Roast Beef Gyro) 1,290 mg

38-Arby's (Reuben) 2,420 mg

39-Newman's Own Light Italian Dressing (serving size-2 tbsp) 240 mg

40-Wish-Bone Fat-Free Italian Dressing (serving size-2 tbsp) 350 mg

41-Kraft Classic Ranch Dressing (serving size-2 tbsp) 290 mg

42-WestSoy Asian Teriyaki Baked Tofu (serving size-1 piece=2 oz.) 240 mg

43-Oscar Mayer Bologna Made with Chicken & Pork (serving size-1 slice=1 oz.) 300 mg

44-Sara Lee French Cream Cheesecake 10" Round (serving size-119 g) 300 mg

45-Linda McCartney's Vegetarian Sausages (serving size-1 link=100 g) 1,400 mg

46-Lean Cuisine Four Cheese Cannelloni (serving size-1 oz.) 690 mg

47-Lean Cuisine Parmesan Crusted Fish (serving size-1 oz.) 540 mg

48-Hamburger Helper (serving size-1 cup=230 g) 818 mg

49-Tombstone Original Veggie Frozen Pizza (serving size-1/4 pizza=149 g) 640 mg

50-Pizza Hut Meat Lover's Pizza (serving size-1 slice) 1,100 mg

51-Domino's Spinach & Feta Hand Tossed Pizza (serving size-1 slice) 610 mg

52-Denny's 55+ Belgian Waffle Slam (serving size-5 oz.) 640 mg

53-Papa John's Bacon Pizza (serving size-1 slice) 960 mg

54-Cracker Barrel Uncle Herschel's Favorite, Sugar Cured Ham (1 serving) 1,180 mg

55-McDonald's Double Bacon Smokehouse Burger (1 burger) 1,920 mg

56-McDonald's Big Mac (1 burger) 950 mg

57-McDonald's Quarter Pounder with Cheese (1 burger) 1,090 mg

58-McDonald's Cheesy Bacon Fries (1 order) 1,330 mg

59-McDonald's Chicken McNuggets (10 pieces) 840 mg

60-McDonald's Filet-O-Fish (1 sandwich) 582 mg

61-McDonald's Vanilla Shake (serving size-1 small) 230 mg

62-McDonald's French Fries (1 order-small) 180 mg

63-Dairy Queen Mini Brownie Cookie Dough Blizzard (serving size-Mini) 220 mg

64-Taco Bell Cheesy Bean and Rice Burrito (1 burrito) 880 mg

65-Taco Bell Shredded Chicken Burrito (1 burrito) 960 mg

66-Taco Bell XXL Grilled Stuft Burrito-Beef (1 burrito) 2,020 mg

67-Dunkin Donuts Plain Bagel (1) 620 mg

68-Dunkin Donuts Plain Croissant (1) 350 mg

69-Dunkin Donuts Protein Muffin (1) 500 mg

70-Red Lobster Admiral's Feast (1 order) 4,050 mg

71-Red Lobster Half Portion Cajun Chicken Linguini Alfredo (½ portion) 1,370 mg

72-Sonic Veggie Burger (serving size-254 g=1 burger) 1,300 mg

73-Popeyes Bonafide Mild Chicken Breast (1 order=157 g) 1,330 mg

74-Olive Garden Grilled Chicken Parmigiana (1 serving) 2,000 mg

75-Olive Garden Herb-Grilled Salmon (1 serving) 570 mg

76-Olive Garden Black Tie Mousse Cake (1 serving) 290 mg

77-Panda Express Kung Pao Chicken (serving size-6.2 oz.) 970 mg

78-Wendy's Triple Barbecue Cheeseburger (1 triple cheeseburger) 1,900 mg

79-Wendy's Grilled Chicken Sandwich (1) 820 mg

80-Wendy's North Pacific Cod Sandwich (1) 990 mg

81-Little Caesars Cheese Extramostbestest Thin Crust Pizza (1/8 pizza=1 slice) 424 mg

82-Boston Market Rotisserie Chicken-Quarter White, No Skin (1 serving=151 g) 480 mg

83-Long John Silver's Crab Cake (1 cake) 590 mg

84-Quiznos Flatbread Southern BBQ Pulled Pork (1 sandwich) 1,210 mg

85-Starbucks 8-Grain Roll (1 roll=128 g) 480 mg

86-Hardee's BFC Angus Thickburger (1 burger) 1,720 mg

87-Quaker Oats Company Cap'n Crunch Cereal (serving size-1 cup) 269 mg

88-Kellogg's Froot Loops Cereal (serving size-1 cup) 150 mg

89-Hormel Foods Skippy Natural Peanut Butter Spread Creamy 1/3 Less Sodium & Sugar (serving size-2 tbsp) 75 mg

90-J. M. Smucker Company Jif Peanut Butter Omega-3 Creamy (serving size-2 tbsp) 135 mg

91-Conagra Brands Peter Pan Natural Just Peanuts Peanut Butter (serving size-2 tbsp) 110 mg

92-Frito-Lay Doritos Nacho Cheese Flavored Tortilla Chips (serving size-1 oz.=about 12 chips) 210 mg

93-Unilever PLC Hellmann's / Best Foods Real Mayonnaise (serving size-1 tbsp=1/2 oz.) 90 mg

94-Tastykake Cupcakes, Cream Filled Buttercream Iced (serving-2 cakes=2.4 oz.) 270 mg

95-Hostess Cupcakes, Frosted Chocolate Cake, Creamy Filling (serving-1=45 g) 210 mg

96-Del Monte Tomato Sauce With Natural Sea Salt (serving-1/4 cup=61 g) 340 mg

97-Hanover Cut Green Beans (canned) (serving size-1/2 cup) 270 mg

98-Goya Black Beans (canned) (serving size-1/2 cup) 410 mg

99-Goya Low Sodium Black Beans (canned) (serving size-1/2 cup) 135 mg

100-Libby's Crispy Sauerkraut (serving size-2 tbsp) 200 mg

The above list could easily have been thousands of pages long. My purpose is to encourage you to think about what you put into your body, in this case, sodium because of its pervasive nature in processed and fast foods. This list is random and based on nothing else other than what struck my fancy. It serves to illustrate not only the amount of sodium in selected foods but also the divergent types of foods to which sodium is added. Strictly from a health perspective, the added sodium is unneeded. Other than stimulating your desensitized taste buds, the only other purpose it serves is to place your health at risk due to overconsumption. The reason I refer to the added sodium culprits as substandard foods is that when healthfully superior alternatives exist, and for the majority of the country they do, the listed foods become just that, substandard. Those serious about their health believe that one of the methods by which foods become substandard is when ingredients are added for reasons other than the maintenance or promotion of health.

Let's consider some of these foods. If you scan the list, you'll notice that it includes some foods hyped as supposedly healthful. These health-boasting tags are easy to spot: *non-dairy, vegan, veggie, gluten-free, reduced-fat, low-fat, light, fat-free, half-portion, grain, natural, omega-3 and sea salt.* Long ago, many fast food chains and restaurants began adding chicken and fish selections to their menus. From a business point of view, this worked out well for these establishments, insomuch as the wisdom of eating red meat has come under more scrutiny in recent years. These restaurants were and continue to ride an economic wave, thanks to popular public perception that chicken and fish and to a lesser degree, pork, are health foods. For this reason, I've included some meals in which these animals are the centerpiece.

You'll find added sodium in an extremely wide range of processed foods such as donuts, cheese, soups, cakes, sauces, spreads, dips, crackers, deli meats, chips, pretzels, nuts, condiments, pizza, burgers, bread, canned vegetables, canned beans, cereals, pancake and waffle mixes, hot dogs, sausages, cake mixes, cookies, protein powders, nut butters, frozen prepared complete meals whether advertised as healthful or not, ethnic foods, jarred foods and so many, many more, too numerous to mention. You'll find added sodium in just about every food, in just about every restaurant, fast food or otherwise you happen to choose.

Prior to becoming adults and not thinking about where their taste for salted foods came from, most children are done a grave disservice, not only by what they're fed by their parents but by what they're fed in the majority of our nation's schools. The kids' taste buds are being trained at school to adapt to a salt craving diet. This will more than likely have negative health consequences for a great many of them in later years as they continue the high sodium consumption diet practiced by the majority, along with other poor nutritional habits practiced by Americans. Many school districts freely publish their menus online. It's an eye-opener to casually scan them, and I encourage you to do so.

There are a few common health food buzzwords or phrases associated with salt that food processors, primarily interested in making a buck, have latched onto. These include *sea salt, kosher salt, pink Himalayan salt* and others. As I stated earlier, salt is necessary for the human body to function, but it's not a health food. All salt, no matter the type, is made up of sodium, chloride and a few trace minerals, which vary in amount depending on the origin of the salt. Table salt is processed to a finer consistency than the others, has most of the trace minerals removed during purification and anti-caking agents added. Kosher salt is more coarse and is not as processed as standard table salt. Himalayan salt comes from salt mines in Pakistan and is pinkish in color due to its mineral content. Sea salt is procured by the evaporation of seawater, and its mineral content may vary depending upon the mineral content of the body of water from which it was extracted. While all the trendy salts differ in texture, grain size and, to some degree color, due to their nominally different trace mineral content, they all overwhelmingly remain sodium and chloride. The difference in mineral composition is inconsequential, and one offers no more health benefit than another. Instead of telling ourselves that we're adding designer salt to our diet to obtain important trace minerals, we would do better to obtain these same minerals by eating the plants in which they naturally occur.

23

Sugar

Let's begin with another of the many misconceptions which so many people harbor when it comes to particular foods. In this case, the idea is that brown sugar is the healthful choice when choosing between it and white sugar. Brown sugar is a soft sucrose sugar whose crystal size exhibits divergence but is usually smaller than white granulated sugar. The reason brown sugar is brown is a result of the presence of molasses, not because it contains fiber. Yes, I've actually had people tell me that brown sugar is good for you because it contains fiber, which we can clearly discern due to the brown coloring of the sugar. Brown sugar is either partially refined or unrefined with some molasses remaining. Brown sugar can also be made by adding molasses to refined white sugar.

White sugar is also a sucrose sugar. Processed white sugar is the most common type of sugar. As with brown sugar, white sugar originates from a variety of plant sources, the two most common being sugar beets and sugar cane. White sugar comes in different grain sizes, from rough to powdery, depending on its application. When comparing brown and white sugar for nutritional purposes, one could technically argue that brown sugar is more healthful than white. One-hundred grams of brown sugar has about 380 calories compared to about 390 calories for white. Equal amounts of these two sugars reveal that brown has a couple fewer grams of carbohydrates and more water content. Neither contains any fat, protein or dietary fiber. White sugar contains some trace minerals and perhaps some vitamin B2 but in such negligible amounts that they're not worth the mention. Brown sugar contains some small amounts of different B vitamins and some trace minerals, most notably calcium, iron, magnesium and potassium. These amounts are greater than those occurring in white sugar, but as with white sugar, the amounts in brown sugar are so insignificant that their presence does not transform it into a healthful sweetener. The detrimental results of consuming brown sugar should not be ignored because the merits of choosing it over white sugar to improve health are monumentally outweighed by the negative health consequences caused by brown sugar. The bottom line is that whether it's brown sugar or white sugar, it comes from sugar cane or sugar beets, it's sugar, which is basically made up of empty, useless, harmful calories. Anyone who justifies the use of brown sugar because of its vitamin and mineral content is delusional and isn't serious about improving their eating habits. Far superior foods can be easily found—think vegetables, fruits, nuts, legumes, seeds and beans—from which the body can extract the required nutrients to sustain and enhance life.

Sugar is energy dense, meaning that it contains many calories and little of anything else. Hence the term "empty calories." If you're going to ingest something, prudence and logic dictate that it should be something that enhances your well-being, not something that detracts from it. Similar to a machine, the human body requires preventive maintenance and proper fuel to keep its numerous systems running at peak performance levels for a long time. Further, like any machine, if not well cared for the human body will break down in a domino effect of failing structures and cease to operate long before its expiration date. In other words, you'll die before your time.

As far as sugar is related to health at its most rudimentary level, who among us does not know that sugar is probably the biggest culprit when it comes to tooth decay? Certain bacteria living in the plaque of the mouth turn sugar into lactic acid, which in high enough amounts on teeth causes them to break down and decompose.

Much time need not go by before we hear yet another news report about the continuing rise of obesity and type II diabetes in Americans of all ages today. This is sobering enough for adults, who can make their own choices for better or worse, but for children it's even more tragic because they aren't in charge. The fact is that they aren't taught proper nutritional habits. As such, many kids don't stand a chance to enjoy a future filled with good health and vitality. It's now commonplace to hear reports about the correlation and one of the likely causalities between the consumption of bad carbohydrates (simple sugars) and the dramatic rise in the last 30 to 40 years in type II diabetes. Sugar is one of the reasons why so many people gain weight in the form of fat. Once your body-fat composition begins to exceed healthful parameters, the potential for all the health problems—many of them deadly—that are associated with excess fat, is firmly in place.

As with sodium, sugar in its various forms is hidden in so many processed foods and beverages. It can be found in canned soups, condiments, dressings, cereals marketed to children as well as adults, canned pork and beans, yogurt, jams and jellies, nut butters, canned chili, soda, iced tea, non-dairy beverages, energy drinks, coffees and of course, in the obvious processed desserts— cakes, candies, cookies, ice cream, frozen yogurts, puddings and some food-like substances that defy my ability to describe them. The only reason I call them food-like is because they contain calories and can be swallowed, which is setting the bar about as low as it can be set when considering whether something qualifies as food or not.

What I find particularly interesting is when food producers add multiple sweeteners to products, as if one were not already enough. One can easily come across processed products with added sugar, fructose and dextrose, for example. Honey, which is sweeter than refined sugar, can be found in concert with refined sugar in a variety of products. And will someone please enlighten me as to why sugar is added to dehydrated pineapple, mango and papaya, which are naturally very sweet? A clear example of screwing up good foods. A practice in which food producers excel. I can only surmise that the same issue is at play here as it is with salt. That is, after having their taste buds bludgeoned into submission after years of eating so many foods infused with massive amounts of sweeteners, Americans may very well require more added sugars just to be able to taste, well, sugar.

The best place from which to get your sugar fix is from fresh fruits. Frozen, unsweetened fruits are a good alternative. Unsweetened canned fruits packed in their own juice or in water, without chemical preservatives such as BHT (butylated hydroxytoluene), which I referred to earlier, and BHA (butylated hydroxyanisole), are acceptable. I can't emphasize enough that you need to read the labels. Make sure you're not buying canned fruit in heavy or light syrup. Unsweetened dried fruits can be a source of both sweetness and nutrients such as fiber, vitamins and minerals but need to be consumed in measured quantities due to their naturally enhanced sugar content as a result of dehydration.

When baking or making desserts at home, the most healthful sweeteners are any one of the following: good quality honey, molasses, real maple syrup, dehydrated dates, real fruit juice, ripe pureed bananas or baby food bananas and other baby food fruits. Everyone's different but usually, once you've been eating properly for two or three months and your taste buds come back to life, they'll reestablish their sensitivity. At this time, you'll be readily capable of discerning sweetness. As a result, you'll be able to cut back on the amount of sweetener called for in even the most healthful of dessert recipes. For example, I've taken healthful recipes that called for 1 cup of maple syrup and instead used ¼ cup. I've sweetened some recipes with only baby food bananas, and they've turned out terrific. When your taste buds are alive, the limited amount of sweetener is more than enough. Even with what I consider to be the more healthful sweeteners, remember, less is better.

For your own health and that of your loved ones, stay away from refined white sugar, brown sugar, HFCS, dextrose, brown sugar syrup, rice syrup, evaporated cane juice, raw sugars such as turbinado, demerara and natural cane sugar. No matter what trendy or catchy name they go by or how they're marketed, they all remain a sugar.

24

Artificial Colors

What are white flour, sugar, HFCS, partially hydrogenated oil and sodium without artificial coloring? No self-respecting processed food producer would serve up one of his delicacies without this essential eye-grabbing ingredient. It's imperative to make the junk look pretty and appealing for the customer.

Food coloring is a substance that's added to food or drink for the purpose of changing or enhancing its color. These colors or dyes are often added to drugs and cosmetics as well. As a consumer you may have noticed a product label affixed to a food, drug or cosmetic package containing an FD&C number. The FD&C stands for food, drugs and cosmetics. The numbers following these letters are applied by the Food and Drug Administration (FDA) to synthetic dyes that do not occur in nature.

At the time of this writing, the United States, through the FDA, had approved and was permitting the following eight artificial colors for use in food:

1- FD&C Blue #1

2- FD&C Blue #2

3- FD&C Green #3

4- FD&C Red #3

5- FD&C Red #40

6- FD&C Yellow #5

7- FD&C Yellow #6

8- Citrus Red #2 (only for coloring orange skins)

Coloring food and the use of color in cosmetics is not a new idea. Humans have been engaged in these practices for thousands of years. In ancient times, coloring was achieved through the use of plant materials such as berries, roots, leaves and tree bark. Certain mineral sources like iron oxide and copper sulfate were considered acceptable by some cultures for use as hair dyes as well as cosmetic applications.

The first synthetic color dyes were discovered in the mid-1800s. They were derivatives of coal-tar which is a consequence of processing coal. In the United States, the federal government first began to examine color additives in the early 1880s. By the turn of the century, many foods, cosmetics and drugs available in the U.S. were being artificially colored. Some coloring methods were benign, while others employed toxins such as lead and mercury. As a result, the federal government realized that to protect public health, laws were necessary to control the use of these coloring agents. Throughout the twentieth century research on artificial colors continued. Based on these scientific studies, new artificial colors were approved for use, others were banned due to health concerns, and some were allowed for interim use until their examinations were finalized. The federal government enacted further laws and amendments regulating the use of these artificial dyes. As research continued, many artificial colors that were initially included on the list of those believed to be safe and as a result were in use in numerous foods, cosmetics and drugs, were later prohibited. Simply stated, many dangerous artificial colors were in widespread use in the U.S. up until the very moment that they were disallowed.

The use of artificial colors has long been a topic of controversy and heated debate, which continues today. How could this not be so when it's revealed that many of them pose a variety of health dangers ranging from allergic rashes to cancer? Many public advocacy organizations have called for all artificial colors to be banned once and for all. The federal government process for permitting a synthetic color to be used is extensive and comprehensive. Yet, in the best of circumstances, we humans can only make decisions based on our current level of knowledge. Things change and at present the thought of using heavy metals or their derivatives for example, as an additive to something that humans would apply topically or ingest, would be ludicrous. Because now we know. But what of that which we are yet to discover?

Artificial colors are divided into three basic groups which are called straight colors, lakes and mixtures. Straight colors are those artificial colors which haven't been mixed with or changed by the addition of other chemicals or substances. Lakes are straight colors to which specific chemicals are added to form a new color. Mixtures are made when one artificial color is altered by the addition of one or more different artificial colors or by the addition of colorless diluting agents. Today these synthetic dyes no longer derive from coal-tar. Instead they are made from petroleum or crude oil because it's cheaper and much cheaper than sourcing natural plant ingredients. Further, the kinds of colors that can be produced in a lab are limitless. New and bright colors are one of the best ways to attract the attention of unsuspecting children to the vast array of processed food products on the market. They also continue to attract adults who carry vestiges of their childhood into adulthood in numerous ways but, particularly where food is concerned.

Artificial colors were used in the past to hide imperfections in food such as food that was spoiling. Today, they are used to enhance the eye appeal of food because people generally eat with their eyes first. Once again society has trained us, in this case, that certain foods must appear a certain way in order to be deemed acceptable. That's why the majority of people have so many inordinately misplaced hangups, idiosyncrasies and affectations regarding food. The issues that should concern them don't register because they're more concerned about the shape of a carrot, the size of an apple or the color brightness of a particular juice.

We have been manipulated and trained to believe that certain foods are desirable while others are not. Very little of this training has had anything to do with the practical health benefits of the food we eat. Humans are predominantly concerned not only with taste but appearance. Color has become a major component of appearance. We've been brainwashed. It's important to realize that artificial colors offer no nutritional benefits whatsoever. They are worthless in this regard. What they do offer is the ability to potentially harm our health, while mesmerizing us with more brightly colored foods.

People are so often illogical and irrational, especially concerning what's edible. We insist on the reddest apple, the orangest orange, the whitest flour, the bluest fake blueberries in cereal, the brightest rainbow of colors in all the junk food we consume. We turn up our noses if these expectations are not realized. We want our healthful foods enhanced and our garbage foods to look a certain way. In America, most people would blanch at the idea of eating insects, which is common in other cultures. Americans are angered by dogs and cats being used as food in other countries, yet think nothing of the unnecessary slaughter, dismemberment and consumption of cows, pigs, chickens, lambs and whatever wild animals happen to be on the "to eat" list. With all of our weird predilections is it not ironic that someone looked at a lobster, crab, crayfish and shrimp and decided that they looked delicious despite their large insect-like appearances? Snails or raw clams on the half-shell aren't the first thing one would envision people to find attractively edible, but they are eaten with gusto. We won't eat something if the color isn't right, but we find these creatures eminently enticing for our dinner plates. People are difficult to figure out at times. Understand that artificial colors serve only the desires of food producers. Have you ever peeled a brightly colored orange only to find the flesh dry and tasteless? Bright colors aren't necessarily an indicator that something is worth eating. Artificial colors do nothing beneficial for you, can harm your health and only add to the other confused ideas you have in your head concerning food. You should be outraged that they are permitted in the food you eat.

25

Chemicals In General

Human beings, in the name of progress and in pursuit of wealth, have exploited, plundered, poisoned and polluted the air which we must all breathe, the limited drinkable water available on earth, the waters from which many take food and enjoy for recreation and the land we live upon. We've even managed to pollute outer space with junk, in the form of thousands of decommissioned and discarded satellites, orbiting the earth in an increasingly precarious obstacle course for any future space vehicles. Most disheartening is that we continue to exploit, plunder, poison and pollute each other and ourselves.

We live in an overpopulated world where we find it necessary to apply dangerous chemical insecticides, fungicides and herbicides to fresh, wholesome produce to ensure greater crop yields. It is a world in which the health promoting idea of organic farming is fraught with adulterations, amendments, loopholes and legalese. This forces one to recognize that what I've been saying all along is blatantly clear—our health is an afterthought.

Processed food producers make what most have come to know as food. In reality, it is food in name only. It is no more than Frankenstein-Food, abominations created in labs which bear no resemblance to kitchens where real food is prepared and enjoyed. These mad scientists would prefer you to eat something that, by way of illustration, looks like pineapple chunks, tastes like pineapple, has the smell and mouth feel of pineapple, yet there is not one iota of real pineapple to be found. And by their logic, why should there be? It's cheaper and less labor intensive to just fake it by creating and using chemicals including artificial colors, to imitate the appearance, color, smell, taste and texture of any food they wish.

We are inundated with chemicals in our daily lives. While it's true that some of them have had an irrefutable positive impact on humanity, some have caused illness and death, and the use of others is questionable at best. We generally cope relatively well with the obvious potentially problematic substances in our medicine cabinets and under our kitchen sinks. But what of other chemicals that most people don't give a thought to, such as those being emitted by the various materials inside your new automobile's passenger compartment? Have you ever pondered what exactly that "new car smell" is?

Depending on how they are manufactured, certain pieces of furniture, some carpeting and even new clothing are treated with chemicals. Formaldehyde is a chemical commonly found in new furniture. The gas it gives off has a strong odor. But formaldehyde is only one of several chemicals that can be found releasing toxic gas into our homes and places of business. New carpeting is a common source of what is referred to as off-gassing. Again, formaldehyde along with other Volatile Organic Compounds (VOCs) break down and spew noxious gasses into our living spaces. Even much of our clothing contains formaldehyde and other chemical substances, such as polyfluoroalkyl and perfluoroalkyl, commonly known as PFAS. Clothes that are stain resistant, waterproof or wrinkle free exhibit these characteristics since they are infused with PFAS during the manufacturing process.

The PFAS in use today are an offshoot of the chemical known as Teflon, developed by Dupont in the 1940s. Yes, the same Teflon used in your cookware to prevent food from sticking until it was discovered that there was a strong link between Teflon and a variety of health concerns. As a result, it was slowly removed from manufacturing practices in America, but some imported products still contain it.

Sometimes we can make a mistake, immediately realize it and take remedial action. Unfortunately, PFAS don't fall into that category. PFAS seemed like a good idea at the time of their discovery. However, after decades of human and environmental exposure we discovered their links to cancer, cardiovascular disease, autoimmune disease and a host of other worrisome health issues. Most humans, even some newborns, have PFAS in their systems. This is only made worse because PFAS, nicknamed "forever chemicals," degrade very slowly, perhaps taking thousands of years to do so. Our drinking water supply has been adversely affected, and these forever chemicals can be found in countless products. It seems that this evil genie won't be stuffed back into his lamp anytime soon. This is only one grave mistake among many.

Some of the thousands of dangerous and questionable chemicals we are exposed to on a daily basis are difficult, if not impossible to avoid. Add to this other hazards including radiation, questions surrounding electromagnetic fields and just too much sun exposure, and it's easy to feel as if we don't stand a chance in the face of this relentless assault by poisons, toxins, particles, liquids, gases and rays. We've made a real mess of things in this regard. It can be very discouraging and frustrating for those who put people before profits. This is especially true while the profits before people giants continue their relentless business of producing harmful products. Protected by armies of corporate lawyers, it often seems an insurmountable task to get these huge companies to capitulate to reason.

Short of locking yourself in an antiseptic cube, you need to live since you're already here. You must be sensible in your behaviors to protect your health. Life is a dangerous proposition and there exist no guarantees for long-term survival, as I mentioned earlier, no matter what you do. The choices you make will fall into whatever your comfort zone happens to allow. What may appear as an unnecessary risk to one individual may be worth the chance for another. Only you know the answer to that.

It's difficult for people to live without having some semblance of control over their lives. Not to mitigate the dangers of living I've touched upon above, for they are real and affect millions of human beings, yet, I'm firmly convinced that we as individuals cause ourselves more damage and suffering by our nutritional habits than do these various threats. Luckily, the one thing we can control is what we choose to eat. Fake food suffused with chemicals is simple to avoid. You can dramatically reduce your exposure to dubious and unquestionably toxic synthetics by changing your diet. This would be a major step in taking back control of something every human has to do to survive—eat. You must decide if it's worth it on a personal level.

26

Weight Loss Obsessed

Our country is obsessed with dieting and weight loss. It seems that a day can't go by without at least one of our media outlets reminding us about the dangers of the obesity epidemic. The alarm has been sounded repeatedly, alerting us to the probability that this present generation of children will be the first to have a shorter life expectancy than their parents. We've been warned again and again about how simply being overweight, not necessarily obese, contributes to the development of diabetes, heart disease, vascular disease, hypertension, stroke and numerous types of cancer. Those already afflicted with underlying health issues, exacerbate their medical conditions by adding unnecessary fat to their ideal body weight, thereby leading to the development of new maladies. The constant bombardment of ghastly statistical numbers along with the percentage of the population dealing with one or more of the aforementioned diseases has left us numb.

In a purported attempt to rescue us from ourselves, mainstream and social media assault us with a seemingly infinite stream of weight loss programs, pills, powders, machines, potions, nutritional secrets, medical procedures, exercises, books, botanicals, expert advice and diet suggestions. Newer and better discoveries that promise the ever-elusive goal of losing unwanted weight pop up like dandelions. You can rest assured that an even better way to lose weight is just over the horizon. All of the commercial weight loss methods employ at least one of these lures: quick results, fun, easy, eat anything you want and no cravings.

It's mostly a fairy tale sprinkled with just enough reality to capture your attention. Regrettably, for them, a large portion of the population buys into the hype because the weight loss industry is a multi-billion dollar per year enterprise in this country. It has the deep pockets needed to keep its ideas front and center. People who want to lose weight are desperate for anything that will make the experience as easy as possible. Remember, humans usually seek the path of least resistance. The only real, logical, rational and effective solution to mainstream weight loss is lifestyle change. Unfortunately, most are loath to embark on this wise path. Instead we waste our money on methods that, at best, offer short term or temporary solutions, squander time discussing, commiserating and complaining about weight loss and lose yet more valuable time seeking quick, painless solutions than actually doing anything meaningful and conclusive about the problem. Although the idea of losing weight is an obsession in America, the reality of losing weight is disregarded.

People are basically weak and undisciplined, especially when it comes to food because they've never been properly educated. Add to the equation bad information, myths, half truths, outright lies and a societally supported attitude that they deserve to eat what they want and it's easy to see why the problem of losing weight is so enormous. When you have a large portion of the population convinced that they deserve to eat anything they crave because they've earned it or it's delicious, traditional, fun or for myriad reasons, many which I've addressed, we are then presented with the perfect recipe for a country of mostly fat unhealthy citizens, no matter how much they claim to want to lose weight.

Societal institutions such as the government and big business (to cite but two examples) worsen the problem by exploiting the weak, foolish citizenry by acting as enablers. The irony is that these very same bodies, who both subtly and overtly promote the unhealthful habits of the masses, champion themselves as their saviors. Our society is structured to encourage weight gain and as a result people are only too eager to give in to their own self-destructive tendencies. Most people seem to be surface-only thinkers. They don't usually exhibit much deep consideration or introspection. Sometimes, people only seem capable of reacting to physical stimuli not unlike one celled organisms. This makes it very easy for so many to become ensnared in the web spun by the systemic machinery that is more invested in obstruction and obfuscation than in the resolution of problems.

When it comes to nutrition, exercise and overall health, there is no denying that lousy ideas consume most of the social oxygen. The bar for wellness has indeed been set very low. However, despite the fact that all these bad players exist who do more to promote themselves than your health, it does not serve as an excuse when you play the fool. It's easy to become a victim when you don't take responsibility for your actions. The populace has allowed and continues to allow a culture to flourish, which makes a mockery out of the high brow phrase so often spoken by politicians, "sanctity of life." This phrase seems to be dusted off and utilized immediately after the lectern is rolled out and a public official seeks to make a political point in the wake of a tragedy or catastrophe. It appears that human life only matters when it's destroyed by something sudden, dramatic, spectacular or repellant. I can only surmise that an insidious public health crisis that continues to worsen every year, which is tantamount to slow suicide, hardly qualifies as being uttered in the same breath as "sanctity of life." Yet, a protracted suicide by horrific lifestyle choices, specifically those concerning food, is exactly what the majority of Americans are engaged in. This, while they continue to obsess about dieting and weight loss. I can only guess that some people don't see it while others just refuse to see it.

How many more times do we need to hear that diets generally don't work? When it comes to going on a diet, what we do is trade a long term solution for a short term gain. The purveyors of diets such as South Beach, Cabbage Soup, No Carb, Low Carb, Fat Free, Paleo, Grapefruit, Atkins, Scarsdale, Master Cleanse, Sleeping Beauty, Jenny Craig, Weight Watchers, Pray Your Weight Away (good luck with that), Liquid, Zone, Blood Type, Subway (yes, the sandwich shop), Nutrisystem, Gluten-Free, Pritikin and even back in the 1920s the Cigarette Diet—instead of eating again, have a smoke instead—and so many, many more, reassure those desperate to lose weight, with words largely manufactured for mass appeal. These people want to believe and need to believe that these diets work. Common sense dictates that if you restrict what you're eating, thus diminishing the number of calories you consume on a daily basis while maintaining your usual level of activity, you'll lose weight. The definition of a diet to most people is that it's a temporary denial of the things they enjoy eating. In this sense, diets are transitory situations. Once the dieter feels that the weight loss goal has been attained, a return to familiar eating habits is almost certainly guaranteed. Also certain is the inevitable regaining of weight, and usually more than what was needed to be lost in the first place. So the diet merry-go-round spins and spins. This is why so many find themselves in the never ending cycle of what is commonly known as yo-yo dieting.

Another problem with diets is that they are dependent upon the beliefs, nutritional and otherwise, of their developers. Some diets eliminate foods that are nearly universally seen as problematic while permitting other foods that are just as bad but not viewed as such by the diet's creators. Further, nearly all diets focus on simply losing weight, not on health. Their proponents seem to take the view that all that matters is the look of the body on the outside, not what's happening on the inside. This is another reason why so many overweight people gravitate towards diets that allow you to eat everything you were eating before the diet began, only less of it. It's clear that diets such as these offer nothing in the way of changing behaviors and habits by educating. What they imply is that it's fine to eat disease promoting food as long as you eat less of it. That seductive word moderation comes to mind again.

If you want to lose weight but only temporarily and that's all you're interested in, then, while I strongly advise against taking such an approach, a trendy diet might be what you'll choose nevertheless. Diet, as in what you eat, not as I've described it here as a popular weight loss tool, should never be addressed as a trend or temporary construct. Diet is one of the most important factors in advancing a healthful way of life. It's not to be taken lightly. What's the point of dieting to lose weight if the diet doesn't address the toxic chemicals it allows you to eat, insinuates that saturated animal fat is fine, espouses that there's nothing wrong with added salt and sugar or says that processed foods are okay once in a while? There is no point because these trendy diets fail to teach proper nutrition and ignore nutritionally caused health issues.

In summary, good health is attained by doing what is necessary within your capabilities. The result will be a healthy body possessing inner and outer wellness. On the contrary, if your only concern is physical appearance, you avoid doing the things that will give you overall health and limit the calories of your poor food choices, you'll probably lose weight, but you won't acquire overall health. Moreover, you'll succeed in poisoning yourself, and eventually, you'll be stricken with the usual array of preventable diseases raging in America. You'll probably succumb before your time because of this superficial regard to overall health. As you lie in repose in an open casket, your ravaged remains will demonstrate that your obsession with weight loss and simply looking good was misguided. The attainment of optimal health is much more than weight loss and what the scale reflects; this is only one aspect of it. Overall wellness requires honesty and discipline, and you know it.

27

Silly Humans

It's tragic when it comes to our most treasured possession, our health, only a small percentage of the population values it with the intensity it deserves. So many take their health for granted until something goes terribly wrong. What a waste it is for those who fail to maximize the positive potential contained within each of us if only we were sent along the correct path. There's a major difference between what we are willing to do and what we are actually capable of doing. There are those individuals who are content with things as they are. That's fine in a static situation, but life is anything but static. Life is unpredictable, fluid and in a constant state of flux. Things change instantly, at times for the worse. Those who claim to be happy as they continue to blithely abuse the only body they'll ever have the privilege of inhabiting, soon feel differently once they're claimed by a disease, more often than not, of their own doing. "It's all fun and games until someone loses an eye," as the saying goes.

As I observe the poor eating and drinking behaviors of silly humans, it is evident that they wrap themselves in a blanket of denial despite knowing the potential harm to their health. Prior to indulging themselves they justify their choices with the hackneyed words and phrases we are all so familiar with. Moderation, treats, comfort food, enjoy, you have to live and, a little bit won't hurt you are the things we so often hear. But does anyone really believe that a diet of fast food and junk food in general, is not going to eventually make them sick? I think most people are in fact aware. Even so, they don't want to have a meaningful discussion about the upsetting part of this reality. Some will acknowledge that a healthful diet is important and then go into a fast food place for a meal. People like this want to be healthy and generally know how to go about it, but their behaviors would lead one to believe that they aren't that interested. Their self-destructive eating and drinking habits routinely encourage inane conversations about how bad they were on the weekend. Many times, the participants of these discussions are the same folks who claim to be shaping up. I suppose it's true that misery does love company as these mutually self-deprecating conversations, basically confessions, play out. They always terminate on that high note, "but it sure was good!" Of course, this final sentiment is predictably punctuated by nervous, shameful laughter.

These people are fools and sound the part. You can be part of that group or not, but you need to make a choice because there is no compromising when it comes to health. Ask yourself these questions and decide. Were you bad? Were you good? Did you have fun stuffing yourself with atrocious foods? Did you get sick? Were you overcome with guilt? Was it worth it? Was it not? Will you take control and begin eating in a healthful way? Will you reject health preferring to eat and drink anything and everything? Are you going to continue to play the moderation game? Will you continue to call yourself a non-drinker because wine with dinner and beer on weekends qualifies you as such? Are you going to continue to seek comfort in speaking with your fellow delusional, excuse making, out-of-shape friends, about the way you abused yourself during the past weekend, while laughing nervously with that look that suggests—what are you going to do? Will you persist in taking part in such inane exchanges as the one I heard in a gym locker room, of all places? It went like this:

Male #1- *Boy I tell you, remember years ago when we were young, the way we were able to drink all that beer?*

Male #2- *Yeah, I remember being in college and drinking beer all night long and it never had a bad effect on me. Now if I have one beer, the next day I really feel like crap. I can't do it anymore.*

Male #1- *Yeah, me neither, makes me feel like shit the next day when I drink but I still drink and enjoy it.*

Male #2- *Yeah, me too.*

This intelligent exchange was subsequently followed by the usual nervous laughter of the participants. Over the years I've been witness to countless conversations similar to this example. You probably have too, but with me it registers on a different level. Conversations about nutrition, fitness and healthful practices are routinely carried out in this tone, as if it's all one big joke. It's so sad for us as a species that verbal exchanges such as this likely occur millions of times per day all over the country. As I was listening to these two guys bantering back and forth, all I could think of was how absolutely moronic they sounded. I also hoped they had no children.

Silliness, ignorance, denial, rationalization and just plain stupidity abound. But it's always more disheartening when you come across these less than ideal human character traits, in places where common sense dictates you would find a greater degree of enlightenment. Conversations

100

between personal trainers and their clients comparing notes about how much alcohol they consumed over the weekend happen with disturbing frequency. Further, some of the dietary advice being dispensed by a number of these trainers is plainly misguided.

I've heard male and female bodybuilders describe how they gorged on simple carbohydrates prior to a competition for the purpose of pumping their muscles and getting more vascular. These same bodybuilders, at the conclusion of the competition, would then stuff themselves with sweets and other junk food as a reward for maintaining their strict, unhealthful pre-contest diets. Part of these pre-contest, bodybuilding diets included a week or two of eating an extremely and dangerously low amount of carbohydrates for the purpose of burning more body fat and forcing excess water from under their skin to expose a greater degree of muscular definition. During the off-season, the body weight of many of these competitors increases by 10 to 50 pounds and more as a result of what they refer to as bulking up. I had many gym acquaintances who were bodybuilders, and it was astonishing and a cause for concern to witness such drastic body transformations in a relatively short period of time. This was magnified by the large number of these individuals who were using steroids and other performance enhancing drugs, often obtained from less than reputable sources. Some of these people were often unrecognizable depending upon what stage of "training" they were in. This type of repeated weight gain and weight loss puts undue stress on the body, especially the heart. The very name "bodybuilder" has such positive connotations. It's ironic that so many bodybuilders appear to be the ultimate specimens and proponents of health when in fact, they usually aren't.

As I've mentioned in previous chapters, registered dieticians, nutritionists, doctors and nurses should be a source of nutritional information and advice, and they ought to serve as models of overall health. They rarely demonstrate this quality because most of them suffer from the same or worse level of poor fitness/health as their clients and patients. Unfortunately, several of these health professionals also share with their clients and patients the similar and inadequate nutritional/fitness habits that destroy health.

Another interesting group that should exhibit exemplary health and vitality in both thought and deed consists of school nurses, health teachers and physical education teachers. Lamentably, since this group is just another representation of society in general, it too is composed of the overweight, non-exercisers, drinkers, junk-food eaters and smokers. Although this group includes individuals with advanced educations, their various degrees don't dispel the typical conversations and ideas they have regarding nutrition, fitness and health. Sadly, this group of silly humans has the responsibility to teach children the value of good health, but they are ineffective. Overall, it's hopeless because most professionals who are in a position to provide helpful fitness/health information are doing an unsatisfactory job.

Apparently, self-abuse is the default setting for most human beings regardless of education, background, position or title. Some are aware of this behavior and others are oblivious. These individuals may practice a few healthful habits, but this is of no consequence because most of their health habits are poor. Very few people have the strength of conviction, motivation, dedication and discipline required to construct a plan to accomplish what is needed to have a healthful existence. This behavior is prevalent in all walks of life.

People display foolish behavior regarding food and nutrition daily. They become perplexed by the huge amount of nutritional information that is available and subject to changes, modifications and amendments. This causes an already overburdened public more confusion. Factoring in that people love to be told what they want to hear creates yet bigger problems. What was healthful yesterday is questioned today, just as what was unhealthful yesterday is touted as beneficial today. A good example of this process is researchers announcing to a mostly food-silly population that alcohol, coffee and chocolate are akin to health foods. This is exactly what the people want to hear. Many who were already indulging in these things have long dreamed of this miraculous moment to justify their consumption. I'm not saying that there are no health benefits from indulging in alcohol, coffee and chocolate. What I believe is that science has been looking way too hard to find health benefits. If you have to look that hard, by my way of thinking, it's not worth the risk. There are better ways to receive the supposed advantages that these three are said to provide.

I've had people tell me that they don't need to do any cardio training in the form of running, swimming, biking or climbing because they are red wine drinkers, and wine is good for the heart, specifically, the resveratrol found in the skin of grapes used to make the wine. Resveratrol is a type of antioxidant which comes from several plant sources, grapes being one of them. It can be found in grape juice, various berries or you could simply eat grapes. I don't recommend the "wine workout."

The antioxidants and flavonoids found in fresh produce aren't needed in your diet if you eat chocolate, right? Wrong. While it's true that chocolate provides some of these nutrients, the chocolate which provides the maximum health benefits is the dark, bitter variety (100% cacao), not the sugary, milk chocolate consumed by most Americans. The chocolate found in Hershey's bars and Kisses, Cadbury, Reese's, Kit Kat, Crunch bars, Snickers, Almond Joy, chocolate bunnies and all the rest aren't going to make the grade by a long shot, so don't kid yourself. In a lame attempt by some confectionery makers to entice a supposedly health conscious public to purchase their products, they've introduced candy bars that boast up to 70% cacao or dark chocolate. What's the other 30%? Junk!

As far as coffee is concerned, this is another of these controversial products that some swear is good for health while others disagree. It's said to be beneficial in preventing diabetes, reducing stroke risk, and limiting cardiovascular diseases, among other health claims. On the other hand, the caffeine in coffee is a stimulant and increases heart rate and blood pressure. It can induce a jittery feeling, nervousness and make sleep difficult. It has been said to worsen diabetes, the exact opposite of what some coffee promoters say. Coffee is acidic and can contribute to gastric issues, including heartburn and acid reflux.

The great effort put forth in attempting to find a smidgen of health benefit in these contentious and widely used products doesn't sit well with me. It sets the wrong tone by endeavoring to show that not much change is required, again, giving the people what they want but don't necessarily need. It's a soft approach that does nothing to wake people up to the reality of what's occurring in this country. It's like advising smokers to keep enjoying their cigarettes because one of the health bonuses is that smoking tends to prevent weight gain.

Those in charge of informing the public about what people need to do in order to maximize their health potential would better serve the public interest if they were brutally honest. The truth is that alcohol (the drinking kind), coffee and adulterated chocolate aren't required for fostering and maintaining a healthful life. The same can be said for animal flesh. It's taken a very long time to reach mainstream America, but it is with far greater frequency that we've begun to hear how a plant-based diet is the most healthful way to eat. Pushing things such as alcohol, coffee and candy-chocolate on a mostly overweight, sick, overmedicated, poorly conditioned, gullible population, which is, for the most part notoriously lazy and undisciplined, just adds more fuel to the fire. The downsides of these unneeded products far outweigh the upsides.

Nothing's perfect but there is no comparable controversy if we were to examine the pros and cons of a diet consisting solely of vegetables, fruits, whole grains, beans, nuts, seeds and legumes. Whether you choose to eat this way or not is your business. The fact remains that the most rational, scientific research is about as certain as it can be that this type of diet is considered the most healthful. We don't have to be manipulated into believing this or use twisted logic to promote it. You're much better off engaging in a vigorous cardio workout to support and strengthen your heart than drinking alcohol to accomplish this goal. Eating fresh produce so that your body can obtain much-needed antioxidants and flavonoids seems to me to be a more prudent method to meet this end, rather than drinking alcohol or eating diluted chocolate bars. Weight training to keep your body fat low and your muscle mass high is a much better way to stave off type II diabetes.

While it's true that you can sustain any of a number of injuries while exercising, and if you're not eating organic plants you run the risk of greater exposure to pesticides, these behaviors are still far superior to not exercising, not eating plants and to drinking alcohol and coffee. If you make a list on a sheet of paper of the pros and cons of eating a plant-based diet combined with cardio and weight training, the pros to this approach to health will far surpass the cons. If you make a similar list for alcohol and coffee, the cons far outweigh the pros no matter how they spin it or you want to see it. The no nonsense, healthiest, most committed people simply do not consume alcohol or coffee. And I'm also referring to mental health because if you need alcohol to relax or coffee to start your day, there's a problem. They are nothing but crutches. Nor do healthy people try to find reasons, excuses and explanations to justify their partaking of these things. Individuals and institutions who support these worthless products cause society more harm than good. To those making an honest effort at navigating their way to excellent health, encouraging them to drink alcohol, coffee and other items in which strained attempts have been made to justify their usefulness is like getting off the highway at the wrong exit. You become lost in a place you don't know while driving aimlessly, in circles, on unknown streets in a vain attempt to find the right road. Wrong messages and suggestions are confusing, yet they are constant and continue to legitimize poor health choices.

Many find it easier to play the part of the fool than to embark on the journey for their best possible health. This is short term thinking and avoidance-type behavior. It is a poor strategy that will more than likely set you up for an extremely difficult and unpleasant future. While it may seem complicated to the uninformed and disinterested, the truth is that leading a healthful life is quite simple if one only takes the time to learn. Unfortunately, too many individuals place an inordinate amount of faith in those people and institutions who, in a perfect world, would actually have our best interests in mind. We are either delusional or ignorant enough to believe or desperately want to believe because we can't face reality. As a result, we embrace double talk, hyperbole, half-truths, lies of omission and full-blown lies.

There are huge amounts of money connected with the consumption of alcohol, coffee and candy-chocolate. A majority of Americans consume at least one of these three if not all of them. It's much easier to spend millions of dollars on studies in order to glean a nugget of positive health news, however tiny it might be, than to keep people from ingesting items that most of them already eat and are unlikely to stop eating. This serves to make those who consume these products a good deal more comfortable. It makes it easy for them to kid themselves into believing that they are doing something beneficial for their health. Most importantly, it keeps the societal boat from rocking and makes sure it continues to sail forth in its usual maladjusted state.

28

Buzzwords

Buzzwords trend. They come, they go. They're like trendy fashions, hairstyles, architecture and home furnishings. What is hot today is ridiculous tomorrow, that is, unless those elite mystical groups which so many are slaves to, and that dictate what's in and what's out, decide to resuscitate something they emphatically declared dead long ago. People are suckers for this nonsense.

What should never be considered trendy are health and fitness. These should be lifelong states of being, maintained with uncompromising devotion. But people, being what they are, have co-opted certain words and phrases while inventing others and injecting them into the wellness lexicon. Some of these phrases and words become badges of honor and sources of pride. They bestow a sense of community to like-minded individuals and sometimes a feeling of superiority to the bearers of a particular label. Think of people who are referred to or refer to themselves as paleo, vegetarian, vegan, meat and potatoes, pescatarian, lacto-ovo or keto, for example. Many people claim to eat "only organic," while others eat "all-natural." A popular buzz phrase these days is "eat clean." I've already mentioned moderation but it bears repeating because so many profess to adhere to a moderation philosophy when it comes to food and drink.

The moderation, clean and all-natural eating designations are virtually meaningless because they are subjective. What is moderate to one person may be an overabundance to another and not nearly enough to yet another fellow. It's a matter of perspective and individual definition. There is no quantitative measure available for moderation. The same goes for eating clean. Who decides what this means? Natural is too broad a term to describe how one eats, although this doesn't stop people from proudly proclaiming that they eat "all-natural." As I touched upon earlier, there are plenty of things that are all-natural that none of us would consider eating. Taken at face value, eating organic sounds very logical. Who in their right mind wants to ingest pesticides, herbicides, fungicides and whatever else contaminates our food? From my point of view, it's prudent to avoid the poisons, but if you're eating organic processed foods that contain added sugar, sodium and saturated or hydrogenated fat, what's the point? Certainly not health.

One can easily be a junk food vegetarian or junk food vegan and do as much harm to their health eating vegetarian and vegan processed foods as eating mainstream processed foods. Meat and potatoes imply that this is the way "real" men eat. I don't believe that it's far-fetched to suppose that the vast majority of these "real" men are most likely overweight, if not obese and suffer from one or more chronic health conditions, probably coronary in nature. The paleo or paleolithic or caveman diet, whichever name you choose, is a manner of eating that is modeled after what stone age people are supposed to have eaten up to about 10,000 years ago and before the development of agriculture. It's based on a hunter-gatherer way of life. It includes fruits, vegetables, seeds and nuts, which I highly recommend, but it also includes meat, of which I'm not in favor. This manner of eating excludes dairy, sugar, salt and alcohol, which I agree with, but it also prohibits legumes and grains, which I disagree with. As with many things in life it has pros and cons. A potential adherent to this way of eating has to personally decide which outweighs which. The keto or ketogenic method of nutrition is a high-fat, low-carbohydrate and sufficient protein eating style. I don't like the high-fat aspect or the low-carb characteristic of this plan. Again, the choice is yours.

There are, no doubt, some people with specific medical conditions who would benefit from one of these "trendy" modes of eating, especially under the guidance of a well-trained nutritional clinician. Remember, these are not the people I'm addressing myself to. Another thing to keep in mind about eating is that trends and buzzwords come and go. The same is true for exercises, workouts and fitness gear. The lost and confused are always looking for the next "can't miss" buzz in exercise or a must-have piece of equipment to solve all their fitness woes. CrossFit, High-intensity interval training (HIIT), group training, combat ropes, wearable fitness tracking technology, kickboxing, hot yoga, Pilates, Zumba, and so much more are all examples of trends. As with the eating methods, each of these also has its ups and downs. It depends upon what your goal is. Mine is health, and that's what I'm attempting to get across to you. Keep it simple; don't allow yourself to be manipulated by buzzwords. Avoid getting sucked into trendy nutrition, exercises, workouts or gear. A simple and well-thought-out plan is usually more sustainable than one that's convoluted or popular at the moment.

29
Faulty Reasoning

Taken at their word, those who decide to take charge of their wellness by beginning an exercise program and improving their diet are making a wise decision. However, the underlying motivation for this decision usually determines the success or failure of the program. In other words, you have to be doing it for the right reason to have it stick. One day, you come to realize that your health is your most valuable possession. As a result of this epiphany, you make a commitment to yourself to improve, maintain and augment your health through nutrition and exercise for as long as you live. This is the right reason. It is the only rationale that will keep you from the pitfalls that have doomed millions to failure after having delved into the realm of wellness.

We come across many of these unfortunates every day. You know them. They are family members, friends, co-workers, casual acquaintances and maybe even you. Utilizing twisted logic, they set misguided goals, which in some cases provided a short-term solution. But health is not about finding a short-term solution; it's a lifelong endeavor. Short term solutions are temporary and result in delayed, often exacerbated, rest of your life issues. Above, I presented the right reason to finally pay attention to your health and fitness. The following are some examples of faulty reasoning.

The New Year's Resolution Crowd- I shake my head in dismay as each January rolls around. Resolutions are a tradition that need to go the way of the dodo. They are as ridiculous as the people who claim that they can't wait for the current year to pass as if the changing of the calendar casts some sort of magic spell that will provide them with good fortune in the upcoming year. What could be more childlike? Among the most trite of New Year's resolutions is the promise to "get into shape." Every January, the newly resolute descend upon thousands of gyms throughout the country, sporting the latest in fashionable gym wear and gym gear, Christmas presents, no doubt. After having eaten their way through the holidays as a grand finale to gluttony, they resolve to leave all that behind.

It becomes a race to each piece of equipment between the longtime, serious practitioners of fitness and the pretenders. The imposters take your favorite treadmill, don't re-rack weights, occupy the locker you've used for years, take forever in the shower and generally have poor gym etiquette. They are merely a short-term nuisance, getting in the way for three or four weeks, only to disappear once again until the following year. These confused and misdirected souls are like one-year cicadas with about a one-month life expectancy.

The Bride And Groom To Be- When their big day arrives, these people want to look their best, especially for pictures and videos that will last a lifetime. It's like playing princess and prince for the day. Lamentably, that's what it is, just for one day. For those who succeed in improving their exterior for this important event, the truth is that their appearance is a sham. It's not founded in reality, nor are the results usually achieved via healthful means. I've known both men and women who were preparing to marry and wanted to improve their physical appearance, commonly by losing weight. Traditionally, however, it's more often than not the bride-to-be who wishes to slim down to appear fabulous in her wedding dress. Not that some men don't have this same attitude when it comes to their wedding day looks in a tuxedo, they do, but this seems to be an issue that more women are sensitive to.

After the wedding? They both, in a matter of time, typically settle into a life of a fat married couple, reliving, ad nauseam, their glorious high-school days on social media. Either they fail to comprehend how this happened to them, or they believe and accept that married life causes couples to become fatties. In most cases, if the wife happens to have children, all bets are off. Forget about any semblance of being in shape. I know women whose "babies" are in college, and they have yet to lose the pregnancy weight, and they never will. In fact, most have gained even more weight. I can only suppose that the ensuing pounds gained by their husbands are a direct result of Couvade syndrome. Look it up.

Summer Looks- How many times have we heard or read that summer is coming and you have to look beach-body ready? Whether it's the advent of summer or you're planning a vacation in a place with a warm climate, you'll be wearing less clothing. This makes it very difficult to hide the consequences of the self-destructive life you've been leading. If it's a beach locale you'll be visiting, chances are that you envision stuffing yourself into a bathing suit, and the idea makes you cringe. If you're like just about everyone else, you sense impending embarrassment and decide, three weeks before your trip, to take action and shape up. Be it weeks before your vacation or weeks before the weather warms sufficiently in your home town compelling you to shed some clothes, realize the illogic of this annual routine.

First of all, you're not going to get into shape in a few weeks. Secondly, this attempt at getting into shape has nothing to do with improving your health. And finally, all your concerns are with the superficial you and your ego. Obviously, you're not happy with your appearance. It should be so much more than that. What are you trying to accomplish? Is your goal to avoid having others look at you and think that you're fat? Are you in search of a prospective mate? Do you want to make others of your gender jealous? Is it that your significant other has a wandering eye, noticing those few who appear to be fit and healthy? And if you succeed in your ill-conceived mission, what then? What happens after the vacation, when summer slips away into autumn? What's the plan? Do you tell yourself that now it doesn't matter what you look like because you can cover your shame in clothing? Do you anticipate with relish that soon it will be time to eat your way through the holidays, causing you to pack on winter fat like a hibernating bear? And when summer and vacation time roll around next year, are you going to go through the same self-delusional process? Why would you settle for this type of existence? Why not challenge yourself, aim high and do something that will truly impact your life for the better? Stop the roller coaster dieting and commit to a healthful life through daily, meaningful exercise and good nutritional habits. You'll be far more healthy, physically as well as mentally, with the added bonus of having a beach-body each day of the year.

Young Men Wishing To "Get Big"- Not exclusively, but it's usually high school and college-age young men who fall into this trap. I grew up with them, trained with them, we "hung out" and spoke often about getting big. It didn't matter how—we just wanted to get big like the monsters in the muscle magazines. Health was the last thing anyone was thinking about. Overall, fitness was a blurry, abstract concept further reduced to ill-advised notions. One such popular belief at the time was that running and cardio training in general, were to be avoided in order to maintain the muscular size gains made as a result of heavy weight lifting.

As with the young guys in days past, many present-day young men and some not-so-young men have this idea in their heads that size gains are made by "bulking up" as a result of consuming tremendous amounts of calories on a daily basis. They are under the misconception that calories are the only thing that matter and it makes no difference where they come from. The key, they believe, is to eat lots of everything indiscriminately, healthful, unhealthful and continually. They want to get big, bulky and muscular, fast. Many do, as a result of consuming enormous amounts of food, and some enhance this caloric onslaught with performance-enhancing drugs (PED) such as anabolic steroids, to name but one category of PED familiar to most.

Even though young men are the predominant abusers of bodybuilding drugs, there is no shortage of women who also engage in this activity. Common sense would dictate that a relatively healthy person taking drugs to alter his physical appearance, as opposed to a sick person taking drugs to alleviate a medical condition, is fraught with potential danger. Many people believe the reward is worth the risk. I knew many people who thought the same thing. Quite a few come to mind as I write this, and remembering them saddens me because they're dead. The individuals I'm thinking about at this very moment were bodybuilding title holders, and among the most imposing physical specimens I've ever met in real life. They were pictures of vitality, musculature, strength and health. They looked magnificent and had, undeniably, gotten "big."

Regretfully, looking healthy is not the same as actually being healthy. That was the one thing they did not achieve, but in actuality, health was never a goal they had in mind. Ironically, the individuals I'm reminiscing about were healthier in their pre-bodybuilding bodies before years of steroid use and its side effects cut them down prematurely. If they could go back in time with the ability to see the future would they make the same choices? I wonder. Health or just the appearance of it? I don't know. I trained with these "monsters," and I use the word monsters out of respect for their determination, drive and dedication to their training regimens. Although the temptation was great and my ego wanted those same results, and quickly, I'm grateful that another side of me realized that they were going down a perilous road I had no desire to chance. I avoided the scourge of PED and chose health and patience. Getting into healthy, top physical condition is not a sprint; it's a marathon. It's a marathon that lasts your entire life. Just as losing weight through shedding excess body fat should be done slowly (no more than approximately 2 pounds per week), gaining lean muscular weight should also be done slowly, but even more so. Gaining 8 to 12 pounds of lean muscle mass in one year, without the aid of drugs, relying only on proper nutrition and correct exercise technique, is the recommended way to approach the sculpting of your body. If you're gaining weight faster than that, chances are good that most of that gained weight is in the form of fat.

On The Prowl- Some people argue that it doesn't matter why you're exercising because the simple fact that you are exercising will yield the same positive results. On the surface of it, I can understand why someone would take this position. It seems to make sense. However, if you analyze this sort of thinking more closely, you can detect the flaws in the reasoning. Most people who are out and about attempting to "hook up," so to speak, want to look their best in order to attract a playmate. These people don't work out or diet because they are interested in their health. They're basically playing the part of a very attractive fishing lure in an attempt to land the catch of the day. Once the "fish" is hooked and reeled in, it's back to business as usual.

People who make themselves look better for the sole purpose of attracting someone are only interested in the superficial. They usually employ any method they can think of in order to give them an edge when they are out on the "hunt," and the competition is formidable. Wacky diets, wackier cleanses, quick weight loss schemes, as well as get buff quick solutions are all methods employed by misguided individuals. These have no place in a healthful life. This is clearly not a commitment to a life of well-being through fitness and proper nutrition.

The Holiday, Party And Weekend Indulgers- An already overweight group that eats and drinks too much during every celebration, in addition to the more than too much they already regularly consume. The problem here is that their regular habits and lack of care have caused these folks to physically deteriorate, usually by gaining body fat. They are overweight as a result with poor body composition, and this is their "normal" state. This abysmal state of being is compounded by the celebratory indulgences, causing even more weight gain to their usual overweight selves. They want to get back to their regular overweight selves. As you can decipher, this sounds like twisted logic at its best. These individuals will live in an endless cycle of misdirected dieting, exercise and partying. They are mostly delusional and will never achieve their best health and fitness.

I Want To Be Skinny- No, you do not want to be skinny. Skinny has its own set of problems. Insufficient consumption of nutrients leads to illnesses such as osteoporosis and anemia, to name but two of a very long list. Skinny people have a lack of musculature, which is not desirable. Skinny people are no more an example of health, fitness and good nutrition than are fat people. Further, the methods usually employed by people wishing to become skinny are, by and large, dangerous to health.

The examples I've briefly outlined above are more about people whose goal it is to give the appearance of fitness and health rather than to actually be as fit and healthy as possible. They all have different motivations for trying their respective incomplete and incompetent versions of what they consider to be getting into shape. All of their versions are ill-conceived, as are all of their motivations. These people will not commit nor adhere to a true wellness lifestyle because they haven't actually bought into the extreme benefits of the concept. Thus, their plans, such as they are, are unsustainable and doomed to failure. You only need to use your imagination or life experiences to come up with other examples of poor reasons and plans for shaping up.

My appeal is to those with the capacity for reasonable thinking. What I'm suggesting is that your goal should be optimal health, fitness and physical development while working within your naturally bestowed genetic parameters. To reiterate an important point, when you attain the most healthful state that you as an individual are capable of attaining and develop your body and its ability to perform to its fullest potential without the aid of chemical enhancements or other artificial means, then you are a success. It's a cliché to say but no less true that you are in competition with no one other than yourself. Don't be pressured, manipulated or shamed into trying to look like someone else. It makes no difference what trend pop culture is pushing at present. Trends come and go. What's coveted today is tomorrow's mullet.

There is only one of you, and that makes you rare. You're unique, and you matter. There are many varieties of precious stones. They are discovered in their rough states then polished. Even once they are polished, they don't all look the same. But the one thing they all have in common is that each is the best version of its individual self. That's the best you can do. Being healthy and fit—the best that you can be—never goes out of style, no matter what anyone says.

30

Rewiring

To truly become as healthy and fit as you possibly can requires you to make significant changes to the way you think and perceive the world. In essence, you need to rewire your brain. The unfit, unhealthy and those not living up to their wellness potential vastly outnumber those who are fit, healthy and embracing their full wellness potential. Let's be honest, just look around. Americans are generally a seething mass of overmedicated, out-of-shape, unhealthy, stressed-out, crutch-seeking individuals who can't wait to get home and plop on the couch in front of the TV with a glass of wine or other alcoholic drink to numb them. That, or lose themselves down the rabbit hole of web surfing.

The starting point when rewiring yourself is to give credence to the belief that your most important possession is your health. The next logical step is that you'll be unwaveringly committed to do what it takes to preserve this most important possession. No half measures because half measures and health don't belong in the same sentence. Optimal health is the goal of rational, logical people. Moderate health is the goal of irrational and illogical individuals. They support this position by their moderate approach in eating, exercise habits and other behaviors. As a result, they never reach their best.

Anyone can attain the objective of becoming the best version of him or herself. You just have to want to. As an individual, once you are as fit and healthy as you can be, all that remains is maintenance. At its inception, this change of thinking and life behaviors may seem daunting. It requires thought, planning, research, discipline and work. The upside is that the more effort you put into this rewiring, the less you'll have to work thinking about it. You eventually go on healthful, full-time autopilot as opposed to unhealthful, full-time autopilot.

Unhealthful autopilot is the default setting of the majority of the population. When they're hungry, they eat just to fill their bellies, the only consideration being taste. When they're thirsty, they drink to slake their thirst; nothing else is contemplated, again, other than taste. The primary reason why junk food, fast food and sugary drinks sell so well is that very few people think about or want to think about what they are putting into their bodies. A clear case of denial in many instances.

Anything worth doing is worth doing well, or don't bother. To realize positive results from something worth achieving usually requires time and effort, again, work. Most of our parents taught us this when we were growing up, and they were right. Nothing has changed as far as this parental lesson of long ago, and it never will. Sacrifice is a common part of the equation. At first, you will feel as if you are sacrificing all your tasty foods and beverages. In a manner of speaking, you are. This toxic junk deserves to be sacrificed. Later you won't feel as if you made any sacrifice at all. Instead you'll realize that you were wandering down a dangerous, self-destructive road and finally made the necessary corrections to get you on the right path toward health.

In a perfect and just world, which we'll never see, politicians, corporate America, policymakers and assorted experts would only have the best interests of the people at heart. All of these authorities would deliver only true, honest health and fitness information. Instead, we are assaulted on a daily basis with health, nutrition and fitness information that is sometimes true, sometimes partially true and sometimes false. Nevertheless, the powers that be always present themselves in the most positive and benevolent light. They push the correct buttons and pull the proper strings in society. With today's out-of-control, runaway freight train that is obesity, those in charge were smart enough to jump on the bandwagon, ostensibly to at least slow down, if not stop, our suicidal love affair with all things food.

The reality is that these people are not interested enough to do anything impactful and significant, which is what our sick nation needs. They are only interested and willing to apply themselves to resolving the obesity plague to the point just prior to rocking the boat. What the majority of them do is spend their time talking about change and improvements in various areas of our food culture. They pay lip service to this food revolution while simultaneously guiding the revolution along at a snail's pace. The absurd, nonsensical changes routinely extolled by leaders are so slow, lame and stupid as far as really solving the problem that it soon becomes vividly clear that these insignificant and toothless policies serve only those who are in charge. The purported changes do nothing more than ensure that those in charge remain in charge. Revolution and change are very scary words to those individuals at the top of the heap. A food revolution of significance would dislodge too many of the wealthy and powerful from their perches. Status quo serves their agendas well, but it's killing you.

There is strength in numbers. Remember, "We the people." If enough of us change our thinking and behaviors and are united in our purpose, then, and only then, will we begin to turn the tide of self-destructive eating, that is, this insidious scourge on our society. If the people lead, the politicians will follow. If we demand and purchase only healthful, life-promoting food, that's what we'll get, and disease-inducing junk will slowly dissolve into insignificance. We need to take charge and force change from the bottom up, not be dictated to from the top down by those whose priorities are wealth and power and consider the well-being of the people only as an afterthought.

Those scattered outposts of food sanity, be they organizations or individuals, need to keep doing what they do—promoting a positive change in the way we view food. Luckily for the masses, change is the only constant. While it may be unpredictable, obstructed, radical, unwelcome by some, subversive, joyous, wanted and needed by others, one thing is certain: it's going to happen no matter how people with competing ideas and goals react to it. In this specific case, despite the fact that so many people can't see the urgent need for a remaking of our food culture, drastic, meaningful and unapologetic change is exactly what's required now. We need much more than the usual underwhelming, symbolic solutions offered by feckless leadership. We demand it because at issue is sickness and health, life and death.

If you're still on the fence as far as changing to a health-promoting brain rewiring, simply ponder why you don't have the desire to be as healthy and fit as possible. Also, question why you lack the will to put forth the required effort to meet this end. If you come up with an answer that supports the position of a less-than-ideal healthy you, and you accept it, then so be it. Best of luck. For those of you who decide that it's time to take control of your own destiny as much as one can, you'll be very satisfied with your choice. Throughout life, our decisions and choices usually place us exactly where we discover we have landed.

Life is work and survival. Every single day. There are big jobs and small jobs whose respective outcomes determine very specific consequences. Let's put aside the salary-paying job that you go to during the work week. Instead, think of the variety of non-paying jobs that are required of you in order for you to lead the most problem-free existence possible. Brushing and flossing your teeth, for example, is a small job, but it's work. You can choose not to practice good oral hygiene, and then you will have to accept the resulting consequences—loss of teeth and gum disease. Many people have done so. If you stop and think about all of life's mundane jobs and the ramifications of doing or not doing them, you begin to see that life is indeed made up of more work than simply your career.

Work and choices. Hang up my clothes or drop them on the floor? Wash the dirty pots or let them pile up in the sink? Gas up the car now, or maybe go a bit longer on fumes? Pay off my credit card or keep adding to the balance? Wear my seat belt or not? Wear a motorcycle helmet when riding or not? Drop out of high school to hang out with my friends or get my diploma? Study for the test or fly by the seat of my pants? Pay my taxes on time or procrastinate? Change the batteries in the smoke detectors, or wait? Look both ways before crossing or simply plunge ahead? Leave the keys in the ignition for just a minute, or take them with me after locking up the car? Eat only health-promoting food or junk? Exercise regularly, sometimes or not at all? As you can surmise, this list of questions barely scratches the surface of the amount of choices we make in our lives and the effort we put into each one. Everything is work; you just have to decide how much of it you're willing to do. Ultimately, it's up to you.

Generally, eating takeout junk food most of the time is faster and more convenient than cooking dinner. So is microwaving a processed meal. A steady diet of this kind may buy you time in the immediate sense but will surely curtail your time in the long run. Even if you're lucky and have a good run despite your convenient but lousy food choices, you will spend the years when you should be enjoying life, unwell and in and out of medical facilities, one appointment following the next. No one gets physically better naturally as they grow older. Systems break down and fail. Your heart, as with other organs, becomes weaker and less efficient. Your lung capacity diminishes. Strength and endurance suffer. Bones weaken. Balance becomes ever more difficult. You can prepare for this and significantly lessen the impact of years of living by taking care of yourself, or you can decide it's too much work to do so.

Why wouldn't you want to be as healthy and fit as possible? Besides mitigating the chances of becoming needlessly ill, by staying strong and full of vitality until the very end, you'd never have to make those hackneyed New Year's resolutions again. You and your significant other would both be in the best shape possible even 40 years after the wedding ceremony, instead of beginning the typical physical decline soon after the reception. You could look forward with satisfaction to warm weather and to vacationing at a beach resort because you'd be bathing-suit ready all year round, having reached this goal through sound planning and intelligent execution. No more packing on the winter hibernation fat for you. Pregnancy weight would be shed in no time. In fact, a pregnant woman being in shape usually results in easier childbirth. Young athletes would gain lean muscle mass the proper, safe and healthful way while learning about and developing good nutrition and exercise habits, benefiting them for a lifetime. You'd have no need or desire to eat harmful food during celebrations or at any other time. Don't get me wrong, you'd eat and eat well, but it would be delicious, healthful food you'd be enjoying, not delicious, unhealthful food.

If you choose to commit to this journey, be advised you shall be part of a very small minority. Many will scorn, ridicule and deride you. You will be perceived as a fanatic, an extremist and as an overall weird person. Some will question your state of mind. These criticisms will be thrust on you by detractors as they all deteriorate before your very eyes. You, on the other hand, while being mocked, will continue to blossom physically as well as mentally. Before long, the naysayers, although many will not admit it, will come to respect, admire and envy you. But that's their business and not your motivation for your wise choices. Your motivation is that you care enough about yourself.

Choosing a healthful way of living will boost your confidence and self-esteem. It causes you to develop a sense of healthful pride, knowing that you have worked to achieve what most people would also like to achieve but what most people are unwilling to work for. Taking control of those aspects of your life that can be controlled will make you feel potent because you will have overcome the tremendous amount of societal obstacles being placed before you on a daily basis. It's a powerfully satisfying feeling to stand unbendingly strong and do the right thing before the very powers that manipulate nearly everyone else with propaganda and place their interests before yours. Rewire your head, and enjoy what living is really like.

31

Exercise Is Fun

Some of the activities that are usually passed off as exercise may indeed be fun. However, when I speak about exercise, I'm not referring to dithering about in the garden or going for a stroll. I'm referring to body and mind-altering manual labor. The fun isn't in the exercise; it's extracted from the results of that exercise. Advertisers treat the public like simpletons by telling them what they want to hear. The message being delivered through shrewd marketing practices and happily received by the gullible is that exercise has to be made into a fun-time activity in order to get it done. The same can be said for so many other unpleasantly perceived activities. Wear this, do this, add this and try that, all to make the experience fun. Do this for fun, do that for fun. Exercise for fun. The subliminal message is that if it's no fun, you're not going to do it. The advertising media treats adults as poor parents treat their spoiled kids. Just give them what they want.

If you, as an adult, buy into this message of manipulation, then you need to grow up emotionally and face reality. Not everything in life is fun. You need to accept and deal with the truth that there are things you must do when you desire a particular outcome. A few paragraphs back, I presented you with some everyday illustrations of activities that are indeed work. Performing or not performing these varied activities including exercise results in specific consequences. If you want positive results, stop prioritizing fun. Only through hard work will you be rewarded with positive results. Success and a job well done are not achieved through fun, magic, hype or gimmicks. If fun is what you seek, you'll be better served by going to an amusement park.

As I've stated, real exercise is manual labor. Meaningful exercise transforms your body at the cellular level. It's uncomfortable, you sweat, you get out of breath, you get sore. One of the main reasons why most people don't work out and why some simply go through the motions is that purposeful exercise hurts. To actually progress and get something out of a training session, whether it's lifting weights, cardio or stretching, one has to break through his/her personal pain barrier and be able to endure the uncomfortable zone for a prescribed period of time. I'm not implying the pain of injury, but the discomfort of lactic acid building up repetition after repetition in working muscles until the target number of reps has been successfully completed in a set. I'm indicating the shortness of breath and fatigue that one experiences as a result of a tough cardio session and the unpleasantness that accompanies the stretching of tight muscles. This is the reality of working

119

out. This is how one exercises with a goal in mind. There isn't much fun to be had if you're exercising this way, but you'll get a blast out of the results.

The people in the gym having fun are those individuals monopolizing a station, who wait 15 minutes between sets when lifting weights while engrossed in their smartphones, scrolling through their emails during these extended breaks. As far as fun goes, the same can be said for many of the folks utilizing cardio equipment such as treadmills, stationary bikes, elliptical machines and such. These people are barely breaking a sweat, and the reason isn't because they're in great shape and exercise is effortless. It's because they're putting greater diligence into reading, watching TV, performing online searches on their smartphones, talking (loudly) on their smartphones or talking (loudly and incessantly) to their neighbor one machine over, who, by the way, is also accomplishing next to nothing by way of exercise. These types will purportedly work out for years with very little if any, positive changes to their levels of fitness and health. I've known many who, despite being gym regulars, actually deteriorated rather than improved. These groups of exercisers having fun are the first ones to brag to their coworkers that they were at the gym. They accomplished very little, but they're not lying.

Don't buy into that line of trite propaganda trying to get you to believe that things that are no fun can be transformed into a pursuit of merrymaking. It's a waste of your valuable time. Focus your efforts on what you want to accomplish. Shedding excessive body fat, building lean muscle, gaining strength, endurance, flexibility and balance, strengthening your heart and lungs, looking as good as you can by reaching your genetic potential, not needing at least a half dozen medications due to completely preventable self-induced illnesses and not dying before your time is truly up, are really a great deal of fun. You get out of it what you put into it. Work smart and work hard.

Remember to be realistic and kind to yourself. I can't stress this enough. Your goal is to become the best version of you, of which there exists only one. Don't compare yourself to bodybuilders, athletes, entertainers or models. It's not fair to you. We aren't all born with a total set of great genes. Also, realize that most of the bodies and faces of the beautiful people you aspire to look like, who are displayed in ads, are airbrushed and/or digitally enhanced.

In addition to the marvels of computer technology employed to make celebrities appear gorgeous, the stars also enlist teams of people for that very purpose. Hairdressers, manicurists, pedicurists, masseuses, makeup artists, wardrobe managers, personal trainers, dietitians, chefs, and, of course, their therapists are all on the payroll. If we had their money, we could also afford to hire an army of specialists who would be paid solely to keep us looking good and staying healthy.

Don't be discouraged; most of the celebrities you see in magazines can't even live up to their unrealistic images presented to the public. Have you ever glanced through one of those supermarket rag sheets while waiting in line to check out? If so, you've seen the photographs of the rich and famous without makeup or in swimsuits frolicking about some exotic beach paradise without the aid of their fat-constricting, lump-reducing, specialized under-gear. They're people like you and me and nothing more than a microcosm of society at large. Remove the veneer of glamour, and you'll see that most of them look as unfit and are as unhealthy as the rest of America. So don't be fooled. Take advantage of whatever Mother Nature provided you with and work with it, not against it. This mission is about you, not them. Reconcile yourself to the fact that your efforts will pay off. Stay determined; the fun will come.

32

Putting It Together

There are many adherents to informal, ersatz health-promoting subgroups. Many of the disciples of these respective and varied congregations often have an attitude which suggests that they alone have discovered and now possess the mystical key to wellness. This causes the ignorant and uninformed a great deal of confusion, in addition to often wasting their precious time by influencing and encouraging them to wander down a path strewn with hype at best and misinformation at worst. These subgroups of supposed health promotion include but are not limited to organic eaters, natural eaters, vegetarians, vegans, runners, weightlifters, yoga practitioners, cyclists, swimmers, bodybuilders, combat sports devotees and many others I need not mention in order to make my point.

Having just read my list of examples of supposed health promoters, I'm sure you're asking yourself why I'm criticizing people engaged in these activities since the criticism seems to be counterintuitive. Further, it appears to contradict everything I've been suggesting you do to this point. Bear with me because my point is a simple one that you will readily grasp. I'm not calling into question any of the activities mentioned above. Quite the opposite. I encourage you to add as many of them as possible to your wholesale fitness and nutrition plan. What I'm referring to are those people who fixate on only one of the numerous components of an overall health-minded way of life and, as such, are convinced that they have the health and fitness angle completely covered.

The essence of a sound wellness plan, from an exercise and nutrition perspective, consists of weight training, cardio-pulmonary training, stretching and balance training. Each one of these types of exercises focuses very specifically on an important and necessary aspect of comprehensive fitness. Combined with a whole food, plant-based diet, they form the foundation for a way of life geared toward fostering, enhancing and maintaining health. These four aspects of fitness, along with this type of diet, are the cake, and any other exercise modes practiced in addition to these become the icing on this cake. In numerous patients, this combination of exercises and nutrition has reversed the progression of many of the self-inflicted diseases so prevalent in our country today. Many of those who were doing harm to themselves due to a way of life devoid of exercise and replete with harmful food have been guided away from the precipice of an unnaturally early demise.

I won't go as far as stating that if you choose to engage in only one of the aforementioned activities, you should cease that activity. I wouldn't advise anyone to suspend a positive habit. However, I will state that if your thought process engenders you to exclusively participate in one of them while neglecting others, minimizing their importance, your beliefs are erroneous because fitness, nutrition and your best overall health consist of a package. That is to say, they encompass many behaviors to achieve the best possible, most advantageous result, with the minimum but most important of these behaviors having been touched upon in the preceding paragraph.

The best health outcomes result from putting together as many health-promoting habits as possible while eliminating as many health-threatening habits as possible. Let me illustrate. I know many people, primarily men, whose go-to health routine is training with weights, and that's the extent of it. Some are relatively strong. However, because they lack cardio training, they are unable to run, bike or climb without quickly getting out of breath. They are also limited in their mobility because they don't follow a stretching routine. As far as balance exercises go, they leave these to tightrope walkers. Not many of them think about sound nutritional practices, and as such, the majority are carrying around excess body fat. I've known some weightlifters who would sometimes take cigarette breaks in the gym parking lot. I'm also acquainted with plenty of cardio enthusiasts who can run and cycle for miles. Their resting heart rates are low, which demonstrates that their hearts are very efficient as a result of their training. The majority of these runners and cyclists have poor muscular strength and a general lack of upper-body muscular development.

There are people who quit smoking, some who quit drinking, some who get 7-9 hours of sleep per night, others who consume a sound vegan diet, some swim, others engage in spin classes. There are a multitude of health-promoting behaviors you can practice, but the key to success is putting the most important ones together. A significant point to remember is that a good exercise program will never upstage a poor diet. Further, one of the most important risk factors for an early death is smoking. Engaging in healthful practices while simultaneously engaging in unhealthful practices is like waging a war within yourself. A war you will ultimately lose.

In recent years, it has become trendy to post online challenges. They vacillate between being simply pointless to stupidly dangerous. I have yet to learn of one which has any redeeming qualities unless you believe that receiving "likes" is the ultimate goal in life. If so, you have my sympathies. How about you challenge yourself to something useful, beneficial and which may keep you from a premature and needless death? Let's call it the *Putting It Together Challenge*. If you aren't interested in maximizing your health potential, embrace being controlled and manipulated, need to do what everyone else is doing because you're afraid to stand alone, depend on what others think of you, thrive on multi-billion dollar corporations taking your money for the privilege of sickening and ultimately killing you and enjoy setting your kids up for illnesses that they didn't have to contract, simply avoid this challenge.

For those of you truly interested in living like your life matters, like you care, like you'd rather do without self-inflicted disease and as if you'd prefer to stretch this thing we call life to its healthful maximum, if you're willing to set out on your own path without compromise, excuses or apologies, then it's you folks I'm going to challenge. The goal is to adopt as many of these behaviors as you can for the rest of your life. The payoff is the peace of mind that comes with knowing you're doing everything possible to live your most healthful life. Your health is better than money.

The following is a list of behaviors I suggest you incorporate into your life in order to do your part to stave off a half-baked, unnecessary, self-induced death. That's the challenge. The more of these habits you adopt, the better off you'll be. What happens after that is out of your hands. Health and time are our most precious possessions. Don't sabotage your health, and don't waste the measured amount of time we're allotted by worrying about something unpleasant happening even if you make wise choices. Something unpleasant is going to happen to all of us sooner or later. Let's try our best to make it later and to actually live until that moment. You may already take part in some of these practices. If so, that's excellent. You have a head start.

Live Like You Care Challenge List

1- Do strength training, also called load-bearing exercise.

2- Do cardio-pulmonary training.

3- Do stretching and balance exercises.

4- Don't smoke or use tobacco products of any kind.

5- Don't vape.

6- Don't drink alcohol of any type.

7- Don't consume caffeine.

8- Don't drink soda, diet or otherwise, sports drinks, energy drinks, juice drinks, sweetened iced teas or any other flavored drink mix such as Kool-Aid and others of its ilk.

9- *Don't eat junk food.*

10- *Do drink water.*

11- *Don't eat fast food.*

12- *Do keep up with routine health screenings and medical maintenance appointments (including dental and eye examinations).*

13- *Don't eat white pasta, white bread, white rice or other refined grains.*

14- *Do eat only whole grains when eating grains.*

15- *Don't eat animals.*

16- *Get your head out of your smartphone, especially when driving.*

17- *Do eat a plant-based diet.*

18- *Don't consume refined sugar (including brown sugar and sugars with fancy names).*

19- *Don't add salt to your food (including trendy sea salt, Himalayan salt or kosher salt).*

20- *Do read labels on all the foods you purchase that contain them, even on foods you're familiar with, because manufacturers are notorious for selling out and adding unhealthful ingredients. They will acquiesce to the lowest common denominator to boost profits. Don't trust them with your health and life. You're responsible for that.*

21- *Don't consume artificial sweeteners.*

22- *Don't consume high fructose corn syrup.*

23- *Don't consume artificial colors.*

24- *Don't consume trans-fats (hydrogenated and partially hydrogenated oils).*

25- *Don't use recreational drugs or medical drugs for recreation.*

26- *Don't use steroids, other performance-enhancing drugs (PED), questionable chemicals or practices for physical augmentation.*

27- *Don't eat any of the processed, usually soy-based and professedly healthful vegan foods, including vegan ham, pepperoni, bologna, turkey, sausages, bacon, hotdogs and cheese. These items are typically loaded with sodium, which many vegans, vegetarians, nutritionists and registered dietitians routinely seem to overlook.*

28- *Do go to bed and get up at about the same time every day while getting 7-9 hours of sleep per night. The body craves a routine of wakefulness and rest and, as a result, will perform better.*

29- *Do eat at about the same times each day. As with sleep, the body will perform better, including regular elimination.*

30- *Do take an active interest in health, nutrition and fitness by reading and doing your own research to keep on top of any new developments. Things change, sometimes for the better, sometimes not. In order to be at your best, you need to stay informed.*

31- *Do prepare your own food and eat at home as often as feasible.*

32- *Do enjoy eating healthful, delicious meals, which may include dessert if you're in the mood, but do so by learning how to cook without using the commonly used ingredients such as salt, sugar, eggs, dairy, lard, oils and hydrogenated fats, which typical people rely on to make food palatable. If you can learn how to cook unhealthful food, you can learn how to cook healthful food.*

33- *Do set a positive example for your children. You are their first and most important teacher.*

34- *Don't sweat the small stuff. A year from now, it won't matter.*

35- *Do something about the big, important stuff. It will change the course of your life.*

36- *Do learn how to tell the difference between small stuff and big stuff.*

37- *Don't worry about what's beyond your control because...well, it's beyond your control.*

38- *Don't care about what people think of you. It's none of your business.*

39- *Don't believe that everything within a health food store or in a large supermarket chain that presents itself as the embodiment of wholesomeness is beneficial or crucial to your well-being.*

40- *Do stand alone when necessary. This is much easier when you have the strength of your convictions.*

41- *Don't do dumb stuff that risks your life needlessly. This would be a book all on its own but I'm sure you can use your imagination to come up with an informative list. Think before you act. You'll be dead soon enough, so don't rush it.*

42- *Do read books, magazines, everything, learning never ceases until you do.*

43- Do appreciate what you have instead of waiting for a catastrophic event to take away all the things you took for granted to make you aware of them.

44- Do treat people the way THEY wish to be treated, not the way you wish to be treated.

45- Do avoid overexposure to the sun no matter what your race or skin tone. We're all human, and all human skin burns and is susceptible to skin cancer.

46- Do avoid tanning beds.

47-Do keep your household cleaning supplies simple by learning about cleaning with things such as white vinegar, baking soda, hydrogen peroxide and lemons, to name a few. This information is very easy to find online. The more exposure you have to chemicals like those found in household cleaners, the more at risk for illness you place yourself and your family.

48- Do keep your personal hygiene and beauty products simple and as free from chemicals as possible. Commercially available soap, shampoo, conditioner, skin cream and toothpaste, for example, can contain chemicals you don't want to slather on your body and, as a result, be absorbed through your pores.

49- Don't, especially if you reside in an area rife with ticks, mow your lawn barefoot or with open shoes.

50- Don't, unless you're walking across the street to the beach, wear flip-flops or other similar footwear in public places such as grocery stores, malls, movie theaters or restaurants. Shit happens all the time and anytime, not only to "them" but to us because we are them. If you have to run away from a dangerous situation, run toward an area of safety, traverse ground strewn with broken glass, twisted, jagged pieces of metal or toxic spillage or fight to defend yourself, wearing flip-flops places you at an extreme disadvantage. Whenever I'm out in public in warmer weather, usually in a supermarket, I always notice that a good number of both men and women are wearing flip-flops. I automatically think to myself that if something bad suddenly happens, they'll be falling all over themselves in a panic.

Obviously, I could go on and on with my challenge list because in order to live like you care, you must first survive. Health, life and survival are intrinsically bound to nutrition, exercise, safety, knowledge and common sense. The challenge list is a basic blueprint for a healthy you. After reading this list you can easily determine that just practicing one or two of the behaviors on it while ignoring the others doesn't quite get the job done. That's not the objective. Instead, see how many of these habits you can add to your life to increase your odds of survival. The odds for a superior outcome increase incrementally the bigger your package of positive behaviors grows. Remember, survive first, then thrive.

Incorporating most or all of the behaviors on the challenge list into your life is not what normal people do. And that is exactly the point. Many normal people would question what a person who adheres to such a way of life might do for fun. I would counter that with my own question. Why is it that so many of the average, normal folks equate fun with self-abuse, recklessness and behaviors that will overwhelmingly lead to suffering and, most likely, an early death? Normal people set the bar for fun too low while, at the same time, deluding themselves and avoiding the harsh realities of their own mortality. That is, until the very last moment when it's just too late. Life is a tenuous enough reality to cope with as it stands. Each of us hangs by a flimsy, fraying string, not knowing when the final fiber that tethers us to this existence will give way, ushering us into nonexistence.

You can have all manner of fun while still learning about and adding more and more life-promoting habits to your existence. If destroying your body is your idea of fun, I would ask you to reconsider your beliefs. Normal people are influenced into the behaviors that harm them by those who profit from normal behaviors. Normal is an advertiser's dream. Healthful, intelligent living is an advertiser's nightmare. Normal is screwed up on numerous fronts and is too busy trying to concoct reasons to convince the weak-minded that alcohol and coffee are miracle health foods, moderation is the key to life, and gardening is exercise. Don't fall for the hype.

If the majority of Americans put it all together and acted in line with the challenge list, obesity rates would plummet, schools would serve only good food as would other institutions, people would discontinue their pursuit of so-called fun through self-harming behaviors, we would eat for the right reason, to nourish ourselves, not for entertainment, sport, out of boredom or for psychological reasons such as comfort. Further, quality of life and life expectancy would increase, people would stop making themselves sick, producers of substandard, illness-promoting food-like products would be forced to make good, nourishing, healthful foods, people would remain full of vitality and stay independent well into their later years because they would cease becoming old before their time. If the majority of citizens truly lived as if they cared, willing to put it all together, their overall well-being would improve dramatically.

If this imagined majority actually embraced its health as the priority that it should be, children who at present are being groomed to develop the same diseases as their elders would at least get a fair chance at a fulfilling life. The pharmaceutical industry, medicine as business and health insurance corporations wouldn't have the ability to hose us with impunity as they do at present. In general, our health, not only as individuals but as a nation, would be greatly enhanced.

You're probably telling yourself that it's impossible for you to adopt all the behaviors on this list. I would ask you what is the point of a challenge list if it's not challenging? The greater part of the population has been existing and acting in a particular way based on deception and faulty reasoning, which have done very little to serve its best interests. As such, countless individuals have experienced much needless suffering. I'm suggesting you try something that should be the norm if so many humans weren't so terribly flawed when it comes to surviving, and there did not exist another group of humans ready, willing and eminently able to take advantage of those flaws. I wouldn't expect anyone to suddenly, overnight, begin practicing every behavior on this list. That would be unrealistic, overwhelming and discouraging. I myself could not wake up tomorrow morning, decide to turn my life around and instantly embrace all the advice listed. It's way too much to take in all at once, especially if you are the type of person who has been slogging along as a result of conducting yourself in a manner opposite to my counsel.

Take heart, for it took you some time to sabotage your health. It logically follows that it will also take you an appropriate amount of time to rise from the ashes of self-destructive living. It all hinges upon your approach and attitude. If you are earnestly ready to embark on a positive life-transforming undertaking, you don't conjure up reasons why you can't do it. You don't quit before you even give yourself the chance to begin. Rather, you think of and focus on all the reasons why you must and can do it. You come up with a sound and reasonable plan. You learn patience and keep your eye on the prize—your best health—while keeping discouraging and negative thoughts at bay.

As with learning, which is a lifelong endeavor, so is it with improving and maintaining your health and fitness. While there are certain basics that remain constant, many of which I've already outlined, there is always another idea or discovery just around the next bend in the road that will further advance your well-being. Keeping an open mind is important, but not jumping on the latest, greatest trending health or fitness idea without fully examining its efficacy is key. More often than not, the basics will serve you well.

I've heard it said that it takes human beings three weeks to start forming a new habit. I've also heard that it takes up to six months. I believe that the amount of time it takes to form a new behavior depends upon the individual. We're all the same, but we're psychologically diverse enough to keep things interesting. However, the one indisputable fact that binds us all together as far as behaviors are concerned is that to change a behavior, the first step toward change must be taken. You need to stop talking about it and simply do it. Step by step.

Pick just one item on the challenge list and commit to it. Don't tell yourself you're going to try to do it because this sets you up for failure right out of the box and further tells me that you are not yet ready to change. Trying is not the same as doing. Practice one behavior until it becomes second nature, part of your routine. Pay no mind to how long it takes you to incorporate the habit, only to the point in time when it is truly part of you, and you are ready to challenge yourself by adding a second habit. And so it will go over time. Some behaviors will take longer than others to stick and that's understandable and acceptable. Don't beat yourself up if the changes aren't happening as quickly as you'd like. This is a marathon, not a sprint. Slow and steady wins this race, which is the race of your life. Consistency is more important than speed.

You may have a preconceived idea in your head as to how far you are willing to go with this pursuit. I strongly urge you to not sell yourself short. If the mind is willing it will drag the body with it if need be. When I began my journey I was hooked on lifting weights. That was it. If someone would have told me at that time that I would shortly add running to my routine, I would have laughed. And to think that I would evolve into a whole grain, plant-eating and non-animal-eating human would have been ludicrous. Yet, here I am. You'll be surprised how your thinking changes along the way. You may adopt positive tendencies that were not initially part of your scheme simply because you didn't believe yourself capable of or lacked the will to appropriate such practices. Start putting it all together to rebuild a more fit and healthier you. Commit and see where your journey leads. No one was ever sorry for having become fit and healthy.

33

Exercise In General

Prior to embarking on an exercise program, clearance from your doctor is a must. Your physician needs to make sure that you have no underlying medical condition that would preclude you from exercising and cause you harm. Once you receive the doctor's blessing, it's time to formulate your workout plan. One of the most important things to remember is that exercise and proper nutrition go hand-in-hand. Exercising without eating properly is as unsound as eating properly without exercising. To maximize your results, it's imperative to do both.

It's never too late to begin an exercise program. All humans can reap benefits no matter how far along they are in years. Of course, the earlier in life you begin the better off you will be in those later years. As I've already mentioned a couple of times, but it bears reinforcing, a good workout program for everyone includes at least these four modes of exercise: load-bearing or weightlifting, cardiovascular or cardiopulmonary (also referred to as aerobics), stretching and balance practice. As we age, we lose strength, cardiac capacity, flexibility, and remember, loss of balance becomes an increasingly important issue.

As with many things in life, realizing the fruits of your workout efforts takes patience. Success will not come overnight for anyone. However, some will begin to see and feel the positive results of their training sooner than others, which is normal. The timeliness of your transformation is dependent upon numerous factors, not the least of which is your level of fitness at the outset of your program. Resist the temptation of comparing your progress with that of anyone else, it's not fair to you. It's trite but true to say that you are in competition with no one but yourself. Your improvement is a personal, individual undertaking. This is true whether you have support or not because when it's all said and done, you are the one who must put in the work. No one can do it for you.

The purpose of exercise is to improve your overall fitness as measured by some of the usual metrics relating to strength, endurance, flexibility and balance. The last thing you want to happen as you begin a fitness routine is to get injured at the very beginning of the program. This is where self-restraint is vital. Remember that it took you years to create your unfit self. As such, it will take an appropriate and reasonable amount of time to rectify the damage. With that thought in mind, you need to understand that you're not going to attempt a 5k run or a 200 lb. bench press during the inception period of your workout routine. Your body will rebel, you will likely injure yourself in the process, and you'll become discouraged and quit.

To avoid these pitfalls you need to train hard but also train smart. There is no better reward to keep you motivated at the beginning than seeing results as soon as possible, even though I just intimated that progress will be slow. This is simple to accomplish by setting realistic and attainable goals instead of goals temporarily out of your reach as a novice exerciser. Instead of failing in your attempt to run a 5k in your first week, you realistically commit to briskly walking 5 minutes away from your house and walking 5 minutes back, four days per week, or roughly every other day. This is by way of example only.

As I've pointed out, different people will begin at different levels of fitness, regardless of exercise experience. I've known some individuals who had never exercised, and 2 minutes out and 2 minutes back was all they could handle for the first two weeks. When they reported this to me, they were quite upset at their ineptitude. What they failed to realize, which I later explained to them, was that they may not have been able to walk briskly for 10 minutes straight, but they had briskly walked 4 minutes on each and every day that was called for in their exercise plan during that two-week period. This was something that none of them had ever accomplished. They had set personal fitness records and displayed a level of will to stick with an exercise program for two weeks straight. Not only were their bodies working to improve but so too were their minds.

They displayed the all important characteristic that is required to succeed in physical transformation: rigorous consistency. When I shared this perspective with them, it boosted their confidence, and they became encouraged. Now, they could build on this achievement. It's important to acknowledge but not to dwell on the things you can't do. Eventually, the undoable become realistic goals. It's far more inspiring, self-assuring and productive to consider what you can do.

You may not be setting any world records, at least not yet, when you first take up exercising. But that's not the purpose at this point of the journey. First, you have to build up your mental as well as your physical capacity. There will always be an amount of weight that you can lift no matter how light. No matter how slow and nominal your pace, you're still moving, right? Your body can gain a range of motion no matter how limited. You can achieve a posture of balance no matter how rudimentary. These individual points of reference are what you will look back on. As you continue to move forward by making gains in your program, you will compare where you are now to where you were then. You'll be pleasantly surprised at your progress.

This is why you should not demean yourself for walking at a slow pace on a non-inclined surface instead of being able to run on it. If you walk consistently, in a few weeks you'll be able to increase your pace by 1/10 mph. This may not seem like much, but each small increment is a personal accomplishment that will make you feel good about yourself. You know what they say about Rome not being built in a day. In time, you'll be jogging, and before you realize what's happening, you'll be running. That 5k race will have turned into a reality.

The same approach goes for lifting weights. You may not be able to bench press half your bodyweight for one repetition, let alone a set of twelve repetitions. A stripped bar may even be too heavy for you. If this is the case, the issue can be easily resolved by utilizing a pair of light dumbbells that you can handle for the appropriate number of repetitions. This is one way to begin building strength towards an eventual bench press. You can use your imagination to conjure up similar scenarios for stretching and balance exercises. I'm sure you can see my point. There is always a place to start, no matter how unfit you may be.

Another issue to consider is that strength, speed, flexibility, and balance, along with everything else, are relative terms. What's heavy today will seem light tomorrow. What is too fast today will be too slow tomorrow. This remains true at all levels of fitness until life naturally begins to take its toll on your aging body. At that point, what was doable yesterday is near impossible today and that's simply the way life goes. No point in fretting over it. Better to deal with it by continuing to train and prepare for advanced age. When you become elderly and are still able to walk unassisted, while your contemporaries, those still with you, are confined to walkers, wheelchairs or their hospital beds, you can at least rejoice in the knowledge that you made some good choices. Every now and then, while training at a public gym, I'll run into an old gym acquaintance. On a couple of occasions, while in the midst of our respective workouts, I've had a couple of them wander over to me and lament, "Remember when we were able to lift heavy?" I usually reply, "I still do, only, this is heavy now."

If you do some research you'll discover many competing ideas along with their reasoning on the preferable times of day to engage in exercise. In an ideal world we would all do what needs to be done at the exact moment in which it needs to be done. As you are well aware, this only happens sometimes because life interferes. In the real world, the time of day you choose to exercise is irrelevant. All that matters is whether or not you exercise each day. Consistency. At this stage of my life, I've exercised during each one of Earth's precious twenty-four hours. My exercise times depended on various factors but were more often than not influenced by my work schedule. This usually required me to awaken at 3:50 am to get my training in prior to beginning my work day. Most nights, I was fortunate enough to get at least seven hours of sleep. Those days are behind me now, but after establishing these habits and keeping such hours for twenty-plus years I became a morning person. Although, since I've become an old retired guy, I sleep a little later now, rising without the need of an alarm clock's startlingly clammer at 4:30 am. Unless you've lived it, you have no idea of the psychological benefits of rolling out of bed when you see 4 something o'clock as opposed to 3 something o'clock on the nightstand.

I find that the best way to start the day is with my workout. By 5:00 am, I'm either lifting weights, running on the treadmill, or peddling my stationary bike, depending on what my daily program requires. I recommend exercising early in the morning because the chances of something interfering with your program are greatly diminished, barring an emergency, of course, because, for the most part, people in your part of the world will not be rolling out of bed for at least another couple of hours. By the time they get moving, you've exercised, showered, dressed, and had breakfast. You will have accomplished more by the time they get up than most of them will accomplish in the entire day. You won't have to spend the day thinking about your job or something unexpected popping up, causing you to miss your workout. Even when you're retired, things can come up; that's why I like this early morning routine. If early morning doesn't work for you, that's okay. The major takeaway here is to make sure you workout each day and at roughly the same time. The body functions more efficiently on a dependable routine.

Another important factor to consider if your desire is to experience the fullest benefits that exercise can afford you is the absolute importance, the urgency, of regular exercise. You need to burn this concept into your consciousness. Exercise is not a hobby, not something that you find the time for. It's not an activity you take lightly or engage in haphazardly. Nor is exercise a leisure time activity. If you understand and believe that your health is of incalculable worth, then you'll comprehend that exercise is something you must do. It's one of the lynch pins of your health regimen. This nonsense about trying to find time for exercise after the kids are dropped off, before dinner is prepared, after work, or before the dog is taken to the vet is nothing more than a bunch of weak excuses made by people who either don't want to exercise or may want to exercise, but not enough to do anything about it. It's a load of empty talk. My earlier advice stands. If you can do it, exercise first thing in the morning before you allow the requirements of your day to derail you. Don't even think about not working out any more than you would think about brushing your teeth, "sometimes," or to put it more bluntly and indelicately, any more than, due to time constraints, you would consider not wiping your backside. First, you exercise: in a gym, at home, wherever. It makes no difference where. Then, you make time for everything else. Yes, exercise is that important.

34

Lifting Weights

Whichever name you choose, lifting weights, strength training, or load-bearing exercise all are essentially the same and geared toward the same general end result, that of building skeletal muscle and improving the strength of the musculoskeletal system. Strength training can be performed using free weights, weight machines in their numerous permutations, resistance bands, appropriately weighted everyday items, or simply your own body weight.

Lifting weights is an anaerobic exercise. Anaerobic, meaning "without oxygen," is the kind of exercise that utilizes your body's glucose stores for energy without the use of oxygen. These activities are predominantly short in duration due to their intense nature, which results in the amount of oxygen demanded by the body to perform the activity being greater than the amount available to sustain the activity. Anaerobic exercises require relatively brief explosions of energy, which is all the body can tolerate when the muscles are being fueled solely by glucose due to oxygen stores being tapped out.

The glucose or sugar stored in your body as a fuel source is employed by muscles engaged in anaerobic exercise through a process called glycolysis. Glycolysis provides the short-term burst of energy needed in the muscles without the use of oxygen. One of the by-products of glycolysis is the build-up of lactic acid in muscles. The lactic acid is what causes the muscles to become sore and exhausted relatively quickly. Regular weight training or anaerobic activities teaches your body to better deal with and eliminate lactic acid, which improves muscular endurance. This means you can perform more repetitions before your muscles become tired and give out.

No matter your gender, lifting weights or some semblance of strength training is absolutely necessary. It's a misguided old idea still held by some that strength is the exclusive dominion of males. This couldn't be further from the reality. Given a choice between being strong or feeble, it stands to reason that all rational humans would opt for strength. I can't conceive of a reason why someone would elect weakness. The very thought of the idea is preposterous to me.

Increased strength in skeletal muscles is the obvious benefit of weight training, yet there are quite a few others. Training with weights builds bone density and bone strength as well. This is good news for everyone, especially for those concerned with developing osteoporosis, which more often afflicts females. Building muscle mass offers protection for your joints. Weightlifting improves metabolism by increasing and helping maintain lean muscle mass and by decreasing body fat. The more muscle mass you carry relative to body fat, the more calories your body burns. Helping to preserve healthful body weight and body composition is another plus. A higher percentage of lean muscle mass, accompanied by only the amount of body fat required to carry out its duties, can help prevent the incidence of the numerous diseases caused by poor body composition, usually manifested by being over-fat.

Strength training improves balance because it strengthens the muscular system, which is one of the systems that we use to keep our balance. This may not seem like such a big deal to young folks until they start experiencing a loss of balance as they become older. It's commonly known that falls related to loss of balance are one of the main causes of injuries in older adults. Your quality of sleep improves as a result of training with weights, which is far better than obtaining sleep benefits from pharmaceuticals. Another plus is the positive boost to your self-confidence and self-worth, two elements central to quality of life.

The human body, when allowed to reach its individual genetic potential through proper training and nutrition, is a beautiful creation to behold. Unfortunately for most people, they have never attempted to realize their physical development potential. They can't envision that they, too, can drastically improve not only their health but their appearance as well. It's common for the greater part of the population to destroy themselves through lack of exercise and horrendous nutritional habits. This is usually done to the point of grotesquely misshaping themselves. There also exist those individuals who may be at what is commonly considered to be a good body weight but have poor to no muscular development to speak of.

To be clear, what I'm referring to here is taking what nature gave you to work with and making the best of it. This serves to improve your health as well as your appearance. Humans look and feel better when they are muscularly developed to their fullest, individual, natural potential. I'm not speaking of those male and female specimens made freakishly large as a result of using steroids or other means that are the antithesis of health. I'm referring to that look, when you see it, you say to yourself, "That person is in good shape."

Due to an enormous amount of misinformation, many women are reluctant to train with weights because they are concerned that they will bulk up. This is not something women need to worry about unless they begin utilizing steroids, male hormones such as testosterone, or other PED. Of course, if you're eating too much, whether you're lifting weights or not, you'll bulk up.

As a woman training with weights, your biological makeup won't allow you to get nearly as large as a man training with weights. What you will achieve by this workout is the ability to sculpt and tone your body so that it shows muscular separation and definition commensurate with the genes bestowed upon you at conception. Essentially, you become a Michelangelo of sorts, with your body serving as the raw material to be sculpted as you so desire. Talk about taking charge and being in control of yourself, this is a terrific way to go about it.

Over the years, numerous women, the untrained as well as the improperly advised, have approached me with questions concerning the commonly problematic areas of the female physique. The main culprits are fat hips, fat lower belly, and fat on the back of the upper arms (area of the triceps muscles). How many times have you seen an out-of-shape woman wave at you as the large, fatty piece of flesh dangling from the back of her upper arm flaps about in the breeze? Weight training, in conjunction with sound eating practices, will address all these issues by reducing body fat and toning and increasing muscle. If you have wider hips, don't hate them; instead, remember to work with what you have. Wider hips don't necessarily correlate to fat hips. These are two entirely different things. One has to do with bone structure, and there's nothing that can be reasonably done to address your perceived issue. Some women have virtually no hips and wish they had what you have. Love what you have and simply work to improve or maintain it. Fat hips can be dealt with as part of enhancing body composition in general.

Some women are at the other extreme of women who don't work out. These are the ones who judge themselves far too harshly and unrealistically, hating themselves for not looking like the centerfolds in male-oriented magazines and aspiring to look like them by any means required. Don't misunderstand me. The centerfold models I'm referring to are lovely, but technically speaking, the most significant factor contributing to their attractiveness is their youth. Airbrushing also helps enhance their looks a great deal. I have no doubt that most of these young ladies are just calorie counters. The preponderance of these magazine queens have no real developed musculature; they're smooth, soft, and weak-looking.

By the time their youth has come and gone, their modeling days long past, most will probably be on the road to becoming typically fat and out of shape. They'll be trying desperately to hang on to those celebrated times by using the usual smoke-and-mirrors approach that most of the population employs. You on the other hand, by incorporating favorable health practices to include weight training, will develop a body that will always appear younger than your actual years. In fact, your body will be biologically younger than your real age. But looks aren't all. You'll also be able to perform better physically and mentally than your untrained peers, regardless of their gender. Further, you'll be in better shape than most women decades younger.

Men who partake in weightlifting and sound nutritional practices will also develop muscular separation and definition in addition to muscular size. Obviously, men have the potential to grow muscularly larger than women because of hormonal differences. Other than that, the benefits are equal.

Proper weight training causes micro tears in muscle fibers. These microscopic tears heal during the days in which these particular muscles are not being trained. On their rest days, so to speak, these worked muscles become just a little bit bigger and stronger. To allow for this growth process, the same muscles should not be worked on back-to-back days as a general rule. Muscles require at least 48 hours of recovery time before they can be safely trained again. In some cases, depending on the individual, more than 48 hours of rest is needed for adequate muscular healing to take place.

Overall, when you train the muscles of your chest, shoulders and your triceps, you are working your pushing muscles. When you train your back and biceps, you're working the pulling group. Leg work is yet another group. Just as you wouldn't train biceps on Monday and again on Tuesday, it stands to reason that it's inadvisable to train biceps on Monday and back on Tuesday. This is because your biceps, being a pulling muscle, are also involved in pulling when performing the usual upper back exercises. This would be the equivalent of training the same muscles on back-to-back days. However, you could exercise your arms 2 days in a row if one day is a biceps workout (pulling) and the next day is a triceps workout (pushing). Similarly, it's not a good idea to train your chest (pushing) on a Monday and triceps (pushing) on a Tuesday.

Of course, there are many nuances to weight training that you discover after some years of experience. Some individuals are fast gainers when it comes to training and developing certain muscles. Others are slow gainers when it comes to particular muscular development. It's common to see people such as these train according to unbalanced schedules. By way of explanation, an easy biceps gainer might train biceps only once per week and his triceps twice during the same period. There are a few ways to increase or decrease the amount of work placed on a muscle group. The muscles can be trained more or less days depending on your needs and goals; sets and/or reps can be added or deleted as can the amount of weight being lifted.

This is by no means a "how to train with weights" guide. There is plenty of good information online, in magazines, and in many well-written and illustrated books on the subject. My intent is to convey the importance of making this exercise mode part of your life and to share some general tips to help you avoid needless mistakes and injury. No matter what combination of days you choose to do your weight training, there are a few other basic considerations to be mindful of in order to extract the most benefit possible from your workouts. One such important examination is to never sacrifice lifting form to move heavier weight than you can safely and properly handle. Men are more often than not guilty of this, although I've seen some women every now and then make the same error in judgement. Too many guys in public gyms, in an attempt to impress those around them or to simply feed their egos, grab dumbbells, load barbells, and attempt to use the entire stack of weights on the machines, all of which are too heavy for them to perform the exercises properly. As a result, they can't maintain proper exercise form, which significantly diminishes the exercise's efficacy, and further, they put themselves at risk for serious injury.

Having trained in dozens of gyms around the country over many years, my own appraisal is that about 75% of the people exercising in these places practice incorrect exercise form and are relatively clueless as to how to lift properly. Most usually learn their techniques by observing the incorrect techniques of their fellow gym members. Seek out a reliable source, do your research, and learn how to handle weights correctly and safely. Remember that your purpose for working out is to benefit and improve your health. Part of this is accomplished through consistent training, not by taking time off from working out and sitting around the house nursing easily avoidable injuries. You aren't in competition with those around you. Leave your ego at the door. When you initially add strength work to your routine, it's far more productive to begin training with light weights, learn correct form, and slowly but steadily progress to heavier weights as your body becomes stronger. This method will also supply a psychological boost because it almost guarantees that you'll make incremental progress, but progress nonetheless, keeping you motivated to continue during those first few months when most people quit.

Not following this strategy will inhibit both your strength gains and your muscular development, causing frustration and disappointment when the results that you expect don't materialize. Improper technique will have you starting out lifting heavier weights, but poorly and unsafely. Instead of progressing to heavier weights, you'll discover that your lifts will decrease.

This is a psychological downer after putting in time and effort, even if that effort is misguided. Becoming seriously injured would be all the more discouraging.

As a beginner in the world of weights and having done your research, you may be confused at the sight of an obviously well-muscled individual performing standing barbell biceps curls using improper form. He appears to be using momentum and engaging other muscles to complete the curl. But he must know what he's doing judging by his muscular development, right? As you continue to learn about exercise and weight training, you'll eventually discover exercises called cheat exercises. These movements are performed by more advanced and experienced lifters in an attempt to pack on additional muscular size or gain additional strength by stressing the muscles more than usual through the implementation of heavier weight than the muscle being trained can handle on its own.

When performing a cheat exercise, for example, standing barbell biceps curls as mentioned above, the primary focus is on the biceps. However, while executing cheat curls, other muscle groups in the back, shoulders, and legs assist the biceps by employing momentum to curl the barbell. All of these muscle groups working in unison allow the lifter to hoist heavier weight than would be possible if the primary muscles being trained were to go at it alone and in strict fashion. What most people don't realize is that even cheat exercises have to be done with proper form, as contradictory as this may sound. Remaining with the cheat version of standing barbell biceps curls as the example, it's imperative to keep the feet planted and the core tight throughout the execution of the curl. Once momentum has assisted the biceps in completing a repetition of the curl, returning to the starting position becomes key. Correct form dictates that one must control the negative (downward) movement of the barbell. One should not allow gravity to quickly pull the bar down to the thighs. Throwing the bar up without control and allowing it to fall back to the starting position in the same, out-of-control manner indicates that the lifter is using too much weight despite the fact that the exercise is a cheat exercise. The negative portion of the exercise, in this case, the cheat curl, is as important a strength and size builder as the positive (upward) movement.

Another common mistake is exercisers performing weight training repetitions as if they are running late and will miss the bus if they don't hurry up. These folks need to slow down, get themselves under control, focus, and adhere to proper form. If the only reason someone can lift a specific amount of weight for a number of prescribed repetitions is because the reps are being done at breakneck speed, then the weight being used is too heavy. Although practitioners of this incorrect form can frequently be seen applying it in virtually all weight training exercises, it most commonly occurs while doing any type of cable-machine lat pulls, pull-ups, and chin-ups. The lifter typically adds insult to injury by shortening the movement, failing to fully extend the arms during the stretching portion of the exercise.

These are the people who, instead of pulling the lat-bar to their collarbones by bending their elbows and engaging the muscles of the upper back and then fully extending their arms to get a good stretch, all while sitting upright, jerk the bar down using their body weight to initiate momentum, while barely bending at the elbows and leaning all the way back. The weight stack can be seen to move up and down, but not because the muscles intended to be worked, in this instance primarily the lats (latissimus dorsi), are actually doing much. This is a waste of valuable time. Exercises, other than during cheating mode or when engaged in other specialized activities, need to be conducted through their full range of motion.

Another thing to be aware of when performing weight exercises employing cable apparatus is to not let the weight stacks slam down. Some lifters use the impetus derived from the little bounce achieved by slamming the weight stack to move the weight. Again, if the weight can't be controlled and the weight stack has to be slammed to perform the repetitions, the weight being used is too heavy. Cable machine exercises do not typically lend themselves to cheat movements, only to bad form.

As far as pull-ups and chin-ups are concerned, one of the same faulty techniques employed during cable machine upper back exercises is also commonly utilized, that of shortening the movement. When performing a pull-up or chin-up, the goal with each rep is to pull the chin over the bar and then, in a controlled fashion, to lower oneself to a nearly dead hang position in preparation for the next rep. What I've mostly seen is guys doing these little half-reps or less. Their chins never come close to the bar, and their elbows barely break 90 degrees. Where's the stretch to the lats, the full extension? People utilizing the pull-up assist machine present in numerous gyms routinely screw up pull-ups and chin-ups despite the fact that they are being assisted by the machine because they are not using enough of an assist. Remember, full extension.

Watching people attempt to execute barbell bench presses is usually a tragicomedy. They almost always load too much weight on the bar, and then a few things begin to happen. Either they don't lower the bar all the way down to their chests (once again cutting the repetition short), or they slam the barbell into their chests, arch their backs, raise their butts off the bench and rise up on the balls of their feet. All this in an effort to complete the repetition. Numerous parts of your anatomy can be seriously damaged by performing bench presses in this most dangerous fashion. Instead, load the bar with a weight that will permit you to lower the bar to your chest while maintaining control, pausing when the bar touches your chest, then pressing the bar up by fully extending the arms. As you are doing this, keep your butt, shoulders, and head in contact with the bench and your feet firmly planted flat on the floor.

Here are a few more lifting tips to keep in mind so you can stay safe and get the most out of your workout: When lifting weights make sure to focus on the muscle or muscles you are training. Control the movement of the weight as opposed to letting the weight control your movement. Full extension is imperative, as a general rule. However, as with most rules there are exceptions, but we don't need to get into a discussion about partial extension weight training techniques at this time. Suffice to say that those movements are best left to advanced lifters. Don't slam the weights. Maintain proper posture throughout the exercise. Do not hold your breath. Breathe naturally.

Finally, especially if you are weight training in a public gym, stop talking. Spending time in most of these facilities makes it quite apparent that they, almost without fail, harbor that element that is there to socialize, not to train seriously. I'm not referring to common human civilities such as, "Good morning." "Are you using that bench?" "Would you like a spot on this set?" or words of encouragement to fire up a training partner who may be attempting a particular personal maximum lift.

I'm indicating the thoughtless individual who displays a lack of common sense by trying to engage you in conversation as you're attempting to eke out that 10th and final rep of barbell squats. This is an inappropriate time, however well-intentioned, to even wish you a good morning, let alone ask you how your weekend was. If you, as the lifter, feel a need to respond and participate in the conversation, then you aren't attending to the task at hand.

Of course, there are also those peculiar parties who, while in the middle of performing their own lifting exercise, feel a need to strike up conversations with passersby, again displaying a thorough absence of attentiveness. The mandibular region muscles of so many of these gym characters unquestionably receive the most attention and, as a result, are the most developed. The other body parts, not so much. Those few who look decent, despite the fact that they run their mouths more than a cage full of magpies, can only be indicative of good genetics, PED, or good luck. It certainly isn't due to rigorous training. It's commonplace to see someone complete a set of prescribed repetitions of a specific exercise and then carry on a twenty-minute conversation before beginning their next set, in what can only be accurately described as *voce fortissimo,* all while occupying the piece of equipment oblivious to anyone else's needs. A good number of the unenlightened actually shout at one another in order to communicate from one side of the gym to the other. I can only surmise that the greater part of these loud, incessant talkers must have been the runts of their respective litters. These types crave attention, try to be noticed, must let everyone know they're around, and that they also need to latch onto a teat. Besides speaking almost nonstop during their supposed workouts, their clamorous voices, in concert with their lack of discretion, gives everyone around them a great deal of insight into their personal lives. People in their proximity know more about their personal business than they would probably want them to know.

Some folks in the gym have a purpose and are on a mission to enhance their health. They go about their business diligently, consistently, and they are eventually rewarded for their labor. Most of the ones who show minimal to no progress, despite years of being members, are the unfocussed conversationalists. It's not that complicated, you get out of it what you put into it. If you have a desire to socialize, save it for the locker room. Once you hit the gym floor, it should be all business. My advice to the chatterboxes is that they should shut up and lift.

35

Cardio

Having read this far, you are well aware that I consider strength training to be an integral part of any well-rounded fitness program. However, your overall well-being is compromised and the importance of how much weight you can lift and your muscularity is diminished if you have a resting heart rate (RHR) equivalent to that of a hummingbird on the wing. Cardiovascular exercise, also known as cardiopulmonary training and aerobic training, includes those exercises that raise your heart rate and can be engaged in for a relatively prolonged period of time without stopping to recuperate, such as running, biking, swimming, cross-country skiing, stair climbing, rowing, brisk walking and skipping rope. Cardio-type exercises can be performed outdoors, indoors, or in a gym environment on equipment that mimics the normal form of the activity. Think treadmills, stationary bikes, elliptical machines, stationary rowers, steppers, revolving stair-climbing machines, and any combination or variant of the aforementioned.

Cardio exercises are known as aerobic exercise, aerobic basically meaning "with oxygen." This type of exercise utilizes oxygen in the blood, pumped by the heart and subsequently delivered to the working muscles, to burn fuel in the form of carbohydrates and fat to keep the muscles working for a sustained period of time. You can see how this is different from anaerobic exercise, such as lifting weights or an all-out sprint of any kind. In these short-term anaerobic activities, your muscles quickly become depleted of energy. Not so with aerobics where the exercise lacks the intensity of anaerobic exercise but makes up for this by being much longer in duration.

As with strength training, aerobics are an absolutely essential component of a well-planned fitness and health regimen. Unfortunately, too many people who engage in aerobics on a relatively regular basis, are not getting the most important benefit from the exercise. This is because they have dumbed cardio down, considering it no more than an activity that simply warms you up for "real" exercise by causing you to break a sweat, or it's just thought of as a calorie burner. While prudent exercisers always warm up prior to exercising, and being aware of calories matters whether your goal is building lean muscle mass or losing excess adipose tissue, the most important purpose of cardio training is to build your heart into a stronger muscle and have it become a more efficient pump. A well-trained heart, having become a proficient pumping machine, moves a greater volume of oxygenated blood through your body. It accomplishes this with less effort, specifically, fewer beats per minute than an untrained heart. The more effectively your heart beats, the lower your resting heart rate.

Aerobic conditioning improves the function of your cardiopulmonary system. Simply put, your heart and lungs work better. This system, when regularly trained, is able to increase the amount of oxygen that is delivered to exercising muscles, which enables them to do more work for a longer period of time without becoming spent.

This concept can be easily understood if you consider the following comparison of two hypothetical athletes. The first athlete is a marathon runner with a highly conditioned cardiopulmonary system as a result of years of aerobic training in the form of running. His consistent workouts have enlarged and strengthened his heart muscle so that it has become extremely efficient at pumping blood throughout his body. The adeptness of his heart's ability to do its work is readily identifiable by examining his RHR, which is approximately 43 beats per minute. Bear in mind that what is generally accepted as a normal RHR, depending on age and level of activity, lies within the 60-100 beats per minute range.

Our second athlete in this comparison is a bodybuilder who has devoted years to rigorous weight training. The hard work and commitment to his craft have paid off and is quite evident by his well-developed physique. His body composition is high in lean muscle mass and low in body fat. He is also relatively strong, capable of a 460-pound bench press. While he sometimes does engage in a bit of cardio activity a couple of days per week, on his off days, as he refers to them, this activity amounts to no more than easy 20-minute walks on the treadmill to burn a few extra calories as he sees fit. This usually happens around the days when he cheats on his diet. An uninformed person who would simply look at him would unquestionably give credence to the notion that our bodybuilder is in great physical condition. But is he really?

No doubt that he has checked off the boxes on a number of the prerequisites for being regarded as a healthy and fit individual. As mentioned, he has a high muscle, low-fat body composition, strength, power and a body exterior developed to its fullest genetic potential. He looks great. His RHR is approximately 76 beats per minute, considered within the norm. For all of his hard work, dedication, and outward appearance of superior physical conditioning, his heart fitness is just average. It's the same as that of most typical citizens walking around anywhere, including many who do no regular exercise and do nothing remarkable.

Realizing that differences in body size and other factors determine the exact amount of blood contained within a human body, imagine that a predetermined amount of blood, let's say 10 pints, which is roughly the amount contained within the body of an adult human, is making a complete circulation inside the respective bodies of our marathoner and our bodybuilder. Again, being aware that body size and other elements dictate exact results, for the purpose of this example, we'll accept that it takes about 1 minute, which is about average, for all the blood contained within the body to be completely circulated.

The marathoner, with his highly conditioned heart, circulates all his body's blood in 43 beats. On the other hand, the bodybuilder, by all appearances the epitome of health and fitness, needs his heart to beat 76 times to pump the same volume of blood during the same period of time. Whose heart is in better shape? Of course, the answer is the heart of the marathoner. His heart has been trained to work more efficiently thereby, it doesn't need to work as hard as the bodybuilder's heart. This is an example where less (beats per minute) is more (healthful) and more (beats per minute) is less (healthful). More is not always better.

Of course, this is an oversimplified synopsis intended only to illustrate the critical nature of having a well-trained heart. Cardiac output (the amount of blood that the heart pumps in 1 minute), stroke volume (the amount of blood the heart pumps each time it beats), heart rate (the number of heart beats per minute), and VO2 max (the maximum amount of oxygen a person can employ during intense aerobic exercise), can all be improved upon. The most significant concept to grasp here is that the only way, from an exercise point of view, to improve these heart functions, thereby improving heart fitness, is to engage in consistent and vigorous aerobic exercises.

I'm obviously an unapologetic proponent of everyone developing their own body to the best of their naturally given ability, along with enhancing their strength. But what's the point of appearing fit and possessing great strength if you can't run a decent mile without the feeling that you're going to drop dead of a massive myocardial infarction? I've seen plenty of big, strong people lift impressive amounts of weight in the gym, only to be humbled by the cardio equipment. The most important muscle you have is your heart, yet most people, especially men, put an inordinate amount of work into building impressive-looking arms, while cardio training is an afterthought. On the rare occasions when they make time for some aerobic work, it's only done for the purpose of burning calories with little consideration, if any, given to heart muscle development.

Lifting weights and strength training, in general, is but one important aspect of a comprehensive approach to exercise. When overall fitness and health are viewed as a single goal, those who strength train alone are making as big a mistake as those who only perform cardio exercises. Lifting weights and cardio training complement one another and must both become habits for one to achieve the optimal wellness outcome desired. Anything else is unacceptable, no matter what anyone tells you.

As with strength training or when beginning any new type of exercise, when you first embark on a cardio program, regardless of your specific aerobic exercise of choice, you must begin at a comfortably easy level of intensity and slowly increase that intensity as your cardiopulmonary system becomes stronger. Remember, too, that even though the emphasis of this type of training is focused on improving heart fitness, if you've never run, rowed, climbed, or used a hand crank aerobics trainer, also known as an upper-body ergometer (for those who don't have use of their legs or those who just prefer peddling with their arms), your body's skeletal muscles will be responsible for moving you through these new exercises. Similar to your cardiopulmonary system, they will also require an adequate period of time to become acclimated to the distinct way in which they are now being pressed into service.

If you are not aerobically fit, having bitten off more than you can chew, your body will let you know. Given your exercise of choice, if the speed is too great, the incline too steep, or the tension excessive, you may experience shortness of breath, dizziness, nausea, or any of a number of other symptoms telling you to ease up. The purpose is not to do cardio until you vomit. The intention, after an adequate warmup, is to elevate your exercise heart rate to approximately 65% to 85% of your maximum heart rate and sustain it at this level for a minimum of 20 minutes. Then, decrease the intensity to cool down and recover before ending the exercise session. The level of intensity required to attain the necessary exercise heart rate percentage in which to gain the most benefit will vary from person to person. It is contingent upon each individual's level of fitness. Some people will be surprised and disappointed to discover that relatively low-intensity aerobics quickly accelerate their heart. This is a wake-up call that should not be taken lightly.

There are various formulas for discerning your maximum heart rate. Your maximum heart rate (MHR) is the highest number of beats per minute (BPM) at which your heart can safely perform during physical exertion. One of the simpler ones is to subtract your age from the number 220. The resulting difference is your approximate maximum heart rate (220 – your age = your maximum heart rate or MHR). I must emphasize "approximate" because no matter which formula you utilize, the results will only be an estimate. However, at least the estimate gives you some parameters within which you can work to help you track and evaluate your cardio fitness. Knowing the MHR percentage level at which you are training is critically important because otherwise, you'll always be performing your cardio exercises in an unknown zone. On some days, you may be in the correct percentage range, and on others, you may be training too hard or not hard enough. This would be equivalent to going to the gym to lift weights and using any weight, sometimes an appropriate amount and at other times too light or too heavy, on your various lifting exercises. It's difficult to track your strength gains in this manner. Another method of evaluating your aerobic progress is to establish a baseline resting heart rate prior to beginning a cardio program. Doing so will allow you to follow the improvement of your resting heart rate as it becomes less. Keep in mind that your maximum heart rate generally depends upon your age, but individuals, even those of the same age, can have variations in their respective maximum heart rates due to fitness levels, body composition, genetics, the environment in which they live and exercise, and other factors. Similar variables can affect your resting heart rate as well.

Using our formula, if you are a 40-year-old, the calculation is: $220 - 40 = 180$ as a MHR. Generally speaking, a 40-year-old's heart can maximally beat up to 180 times per minute. As we become older, our maximum heart rate lessens. An 18-year-old's heart can beat up to 202 times per minute, $220 - 18 = 202$, while a 70-year-old heart can only beat a maximum of 150 times per minute, $220 - 70 = 150$. Don't examine these numbers and assume that an 18-year-old is going to automatically be much more fit than a 70-year-old just because the 70-year-old's heart can only beat 150 times per minute. This is not necessarily the case, especially if we are looking at a fit 70-year-old and an unfit 18-year-old.

A strong and efficient heart is obviously vital at any age, but perhaps more so if we are fortunate enough to attain old age. The better your heart functions, the less it needs to work to deliver life-sustaining oxygen by way of your blood to your body's numerous components. Further, I think we can all agree that stress is an unfortunate part of life. A strong heart is better able to cope with stress.

Since we spend more time each day resting per se, as opposed to performing cardiopulmonary exercises with our exercise heart rates in the proper training zone, it's essential that when it's time for our cardio session, we put effort and intensity into this training. Within the structure of a well-thought-out workout routine, the heart must be pushed and trained like other muscles so that the daily rigors of living don't always send it into a frenzy of rapid beating. Walking about, climbing a short flight of stairs, rising out of a chair, or bending over to pick something off the floor shouldn't have your heart thumping in your chest as if you were attempting to break the world record in the 100-meter sprint. Unfortunately, for so many, this is exactly the case.

Now, I'm not referring to the type of cardio I usually encounter at the numerous gyms in which I've trained. Most of the people I see doing cardio at the gym should just stay home for what they are accomplishing. I see them occupying all sorts of cardio equipment, and without fail, the majority are talking to someone next to them, across from them, or shouting to someone on the gym floor. I see and hear them laughing, reading newspapers, magazines, and books. They're speaking on their smartphones, web-surfing or checking emails. Those in the minority are the ones training in an intense, focused manner while trying to ignore the foolishness taking place around them. When a person is working at a maximum level of intensity while engaged in a cardio activity, he is in his own personal hell sucking wind, muscles on fire, and counting down the minutes until it's over. His purpose is to improve his overall fitness and health which will hopefully extend his chances of survivability. The last thing he needs from this world that does so much to diminish anyone's chance of an extended stay, is for some ignoramus to hop onto the machine right next to him and begin to yuk it up on his phone or laugh hysterically at some stupidity with the other imbecile next to him. This inconsiderate and disruptive behavior occurring in such close proximity to the person actually exercising, makes his task that much more difficult.

Of course the fools can chat and laugh. They're, and I'm using the word loosely here, "exercising," at level 1 and not because they're new to the gym. They've been coming here for years, but you wouldn't know it by looking at them. They've wasted a good portion of their lives telling themselves and all their friends that they go to the gym, which they do, but progress escapes their meager efforts. They're moving so slowly they are barely moving at all. Yet, they maintain a death grip on the machine, which brings me to another point.

When using certain step climbing machines, steppers, elliptical trainers, and similar equipment, it is advisable to lightly grasp the respective machine in the place provided to maintain balance and stability. This is particularly important if one is moving at a relatively fast pace. This is a safety issue. However, if you are walking or running on a treadmill, you should not be holding on unless you're recovering from an illness that compromises your balance. When you hold on, you're not expending as much of an effort as you think. Pay no mind to the caloric readout after a session of holding on. The calories displayed are the approximate calories you would have burned had you not been holding on. As a rule, even if you're not holding on, these are estimates of calories burned, not hard and fast numbers.

Additionally, where calorie displays are concerned, many people have the mistaken impression that the readout shown on any given piece of cardio equipment at the end of a workout represents a total of "extra" calories burned to be tacked onto the daily total of calories burned. This is incorrect. These calories are simply an estimated representation of calories burned during the exercise session. Let's say, for the sake of discussion, that the number is 350 (calories) expended in 30 minutes of aerobics. Had you not been exercising and instead, had you been sitting on the couch reading a book, you would have, nonetheless, been burning calories. Not as many as during the workout but still burning them. Again, for the sake of discussion, we'll guesstimate that while you were reading, you expended 50 calories. My point is that the mere act of being alive burns calories, even during sleep. It just depends upon what you are doing during a given period of time that will determine exactly how many calories you use up. So, you didn't burn 350 "extra" calories, simply 350 calories because that's what you were doing for that particular 30 minutes of your day. Obviously, the more active you are, the more calories you'll burn, but forget the term "extra."

Another observation which I've made countless times is one that serves as the antithesis of the individuals laughing it up and barely moving on their treadmills. In this case, it's those few individuals running at such a high rate of speed, as if their hair were on fire, and holding on as if their very lives depended on it (because they literally do). These misguided souls actually believe they are running at the break-neck pace that they have entered into the machine. They aren't. It's painfully obvious because the belt is revolving with far greater speed than their legs can move. That's why these individuals hang on. They spend most of the session with both their legs suspended in midair like Hermes or a flag held taught in a gale-force wind while the treadmill's belt rotates at blazing speed. At that belt speed, if they were to let go, they'd be jettisoned backward like a missile and crash right through the gym's plate glass window and out into the parking lot. Know your limitations and be honest with yourself before you get hurt.

This next piece of advice is for those using the stair climbing machines. Stand upright. Too many people drape themselves over the top of the machine and support most of their weight on their forearms. There is no cheat method for utilizing a stair climber. You either have good form, or you don't. The more your form suffers, the less you get from the exercise. As with weight training, cardio training requires concentration, focus, and form. Cardio similarly dictates that you start out easy and make it progressively harder as your conditioning improves. Again, leave your ego at the door. You're only opponent is you. Your aerobic workouts serve to improve your fitness and health, not to impress anyone. Be patient, train hard, train smart, and please, stop talking.

36

Stretching

Stretching is one of the most neglected exercises, and as with cardio, many have trivialized it. For a good number of exercisers, a few seconds of quick, bouncy movements prior to a weight training session or a long run is all there is to it. For others it's simply an afterthought, if thought of at all. The reality is that stretching is on par with strength training and aerobics if we're talking about essential exercises. When muscles are repeatedly used during daily activities and especially during structured exercise, they become shortened or what is usually referred to as "tight." Muscles need to be stretched with the same dedication and regularity that is given to weight training and cardio but even more often, as in every day.

Prior to exercise, stretching improves range of motion or "flexibility," as it's commonly called. This reduces the chances of injury not only when training but also while carrying out life's mundane chores. The better range of motion you have, the less chance there is of you experiencing an overextension injury or a muscular strain type injury due to a simple, routine movement inside or outside of the gym that would be of no consequence if you had good flexibility. After exercise, engaging in movements that enhance muscular elasticity helps diminish the muscle and joint soreness associated post-workout by relaxing muscles and counteracting the muscle-shortening effects of exercise.

With improved flexibility comes improved functionality and proficiency of movement by requiring less power to extend your range of motion. Stretching also improves posture, especially stretches involving the hamstrings, quadriceps, hips, lower back, shoulders and chest. Improved posture through stretching can relieve lower back pain. Flexibility exercises promote superior blood supply to muscles and joints. Greater blood supply makes for an improved nutrient delivery system. Additionally, tight muscles under a constant state of tension can cause mental stress. Relaxing the muscles can relax the mind. Stretching can also help promote a better sense of overall balance due to the resultant muscular flexibility, creating fluidity and greater ease of movement.

Some people believe in static stretching—holding a position for a prescribed period of time, typically 30 to 60 seconds—prior to exercise. I disagree because the static stretching of a cold, tight muscle seems to me like a recipe for, at the very least, a pulled muscle. Instead, I am a proponent of warming up a muscle prior to exercise by incorporating dynamic stretching—slow, light, deliberate movements through a specific range of motion—which encourages more blood flow to the area about to be worked. I believe it makes more sense to stretch statically after a workout despite the fact that the muscle has been shortened by exercise because, at this time, the muscle is warm. There are differences of opinion when it comes to this. Experiment and see which technique works best for you. The bottom line is to make sure you stretch.

After a workout, a flexibility session functions as both a mental and a physical cool-down period. Weight training and aerobics tighten muscles which are then more prone to injury. If you've ever experienced a pulled or strained hamstring, calf muscle, Achilles tendon, groin, pectoral muscle, or muscle spasms as the result of a tight lower back, then you know exactly what I'm getting at. The key here is prevention of injury. We stretch both statically and dynamically to mitigate the chances that we will rip, tear, or pull a muscle. Stretching is not something that you wait to do until you get hurt. Stretching is imperative.

As with weight training and cardio, stretching requires patience, concentration, focus, and form in order to improve your ability. A muscle should be statically and dynamically stretched to the point of mild discomfort, not pain. The static stretch should be held for at least a slow count of 10, as a general rule. My experience has shown that certain individual's specific muscles, such as hamstrings for example, respond more favorably to a count of 30 when being stretched. The dynamic stretch should be performed in sets of 10-15 repetitions. The main thing to remember is to move gently and slowly into both types of stretches while considering your ability, range of motion, and your other body specific characteristics. Avoid jerky, bouncy, and rapid ballistic movements. Lose yourself in the stretch—focus. As was discussed when addressing strength training and aerobics, you cannot breathe properly and achieve an adequate stretching workout if you're laughing it up, chatting, checking emails, or doing anything but stretching. If you watch a serious yoga practitioner go through poses, which are, in essence, stretches, you will observe that the individual appears lost in what he is doing, breathing deeply and evenly, calm, focused, and distracted by nothing. This is how you stretch.

One of the things that makes stretching satisfying is that you can set goals and gauge your progress as you advance toward them, just as you can with your strength and cardio training. Perhaps one of your strength goals is to bench press or squat a certain weight. Maybe one of your cardio goals is to run a 5k race within a specified time. If you apply similarly appropriate goals to your stretch routine, these will make stretching that much more enjoyable and productive. As an example, while standing up straight, can you bend at the waist while keeping your knees almost locked (soft knees) and place your palms flat on the floor? While sitting on the floor with your legs straight out in front of you, can you reach and touch your toes or touch your forehead to your knees? If you can't even come close to performing any of these stretches, then you have something to shoot for, provided your body is structurally capable. You can only do your best, and isn't that what we're talking about?

There are a variety of stretching exercises or movements that can be employed to work the same muscle. Some may work better for you than others as far as practicality of movement due to possible bodily restrictions. Try different stretches for the same muscle and see which you prefer. This book is not meant to be a stretching manual, and it's not my intent to inundate you with all the nuances of stretching. You can easily pick up a stretching book or check the numerous websites and observe the multitude of stretching possibilities. See where you stand. How close can you come to the range of motion depicted in the examples? With perseverance, consistency, and a well-defined orientation to the task at hand, you will improve and reach your potential. Listen to your body so as not to overstretch and strain a muscle. Remember to work at your own pace and that there's a difference between tolerable discomfort and real pain.

37

Balance

If cardio and flexibility exercises have been relegated to second-class citizen status by so many who take part in some manner of exercise, then balance training doesn't even register on the vast majority of anyone's radar, exercisers or not. This is unfortunate because balance, not unlike our other physical attributes, begins to decline in our advanced years. How many times have you heard of an elder falling as a result of losing his or her balance, breaking a hip, being hospitalized, and then dying of pneumonia while still in the hospital recovering from the hip fracture? It's become a dark humor cliché.

Our sense of balance is the result of an intricate assemblage of different bodily systems working in tandem, which lets our brain know where our body is relative to our surroundings. Another way of explaining balance is to say that it's the body's ability to sustain its center of gravity over its supporting base. In order to maintain our balance, the four primary systems which must cooperate are the visual, vestibular, muscular, and somatosensory systems.

The visual system, how we use our eyes to receive information from the outside world, which is then transferred to the brain, allows us to perceive whether we are upright, upside down, or in any other spatial orientation. It lets us know if we, or our surroundings, are moving and, if so, in which direction. If vision is compromised in any way, it could adversely affect one's ability to maintain a good sense of balance and steadiness. Maintaining good eye health is essential in general and for supporting a solid sense of balance in particular. Routine medical procedures should include regularly scheduled eye exams.

The vestibular sensory system is made up of the components of the inner ear. It is a structure that provides input to the brain relating to balance, motion, and again, spatial orientation in whichever environment we occupy. It permits us to coordinate our body movements with balance. I'm sure you've heard of people with inner ear infections sometimes experiencing vertigo, the nauseating and dizzying feeling that they are spinning, or that things around them are spinning, causing a loss of balance and coordination.

The musculoskeletal system allows the body to make appropriate adjustments in order to maintain balance in response to environmental instability. Strong muscles allow the body, or specific parts of the body, to make the required adaptations in space in an easy and efficient manner when signaled to do so by sense organs embedded therein. Muscles atrophied and weakened as a result of desuetude cannot effectively perform the work required of them to ensure the body's stability.

The somatosensory system, to explain it in its simplest terms, has to do with our nuanced sense of feel, which is to say, those sensations such as touch, vibration, pain, pressure, itch, temperature, body position, and the like. Particular nerve endings in our skin help the brain identify the nature of the surface on or in which the body is stationary or on or in which the body is moving. As a result of the information delivered to the brain via neural pathways, our skeletal muscles are able to respond congruently to the wide variety of superficies on which we can find ourselves balancing, whether statically or in a state of motion, such as ice, sand, grass or a hardwood floor, to name but a handful.

As we age, balance becomes increasingly more difficult for a number of reasons, including the loss of muscular strength, flexibility, and stamina. A relatively good sense of balance can be maintained, and a dramatic loss of bodily stability need not occur if we work on it through suitable exercises, in the same way, we work to improve and maintain our strength, endurance, and flexibility. We are, to a high degree, in control of preserving our sense of balance if we so choose. The more fit and healthy we are, the better sense of balance we will have. If you've abused your body by engaging in detrimental behaviors such as not exercising, eating junk food, smoking, drinking, and drugging, to name but a few of the ways in which humans practice self-destruction, you have cultivated an environment in which disease and injury can easily take root.

Specific balance exercises can be as simple as trying to stand on one foot for a specified time, 15 seconds, for example, by just lifting the other foot a couple of inches off the floor. If you're really unstable, be sure to have a chair, table, countertop, or other solid object in front of you and within reach to grab onto if you feel yourself about to topple over. You can make this exercise more difficult by raising your knee as high as possible while balancing on one foot. Try variations such as wrapping your arms around the raised knee or raising the knee while holding your arms out horizontally to the floor.

All balance exercises, including something as simple as raising your foot a couple of inches off of the floor, can be made much more challenging by simply closing your eyes. Try it and see for yourself. You'll begin to appreciate what an integral part the visual system plays in your ability to remain stable. Use your imagination for discovering and working on different balance positions. As with all other exercises, do some research, read articles and books on improving balance, and search online.

38

No Food Is Perfect

We all need to admit to the fact that no food or beverage is absolutely perfect. It must then follow that none of the numerous dietary methodologies or gastronomical habits that humans practice are perfect. This holds true whether your choice of eating is organic, natural, vegetarian, vegan, macrobiotic, flexitarian, meat and potatoes, or anything that will fit into your mouth. Each eating practice and type of food has its upsides and downsides. This is why people have so many disagreements about the way they choose to eat and about each food's individual health benefits or not. To be clear, I'm speaking about the eating habits of those people generally regarded as healthy, not individuals with dietary needs and restrictions based on medical conditions beyond their control. There are no "superfoods," "miracle foods," or "super nutrients." There is only hype and reality.

Take the case of water, arguably the most essential nutrient we consume even though it provides us with no nutritional calories. Our very bodies are composed mostly of water, averaging about 60%, but can vary from about 45% - 75%, depending on gender, age, body size, and body composition, filling all the spaces between our cells. All of the body's biochemical reactions occur in a water environment. Typically, without consuming water in one form or another, we would become dehydrated and might last about a week, depending on the individual, before we would eventually die. It's actually an understatement to say that water is very important to our health. However, there is such a thing as drinking too much water, and although it's uncommon, especially when compared to the large number of people who don't drink enough water, the condition known as hyponatremia or water intoxication is potentially life-threatening. Drinking too much water can dilute the sodium in our blood and throw off the body's delicate electrolyte balance by diminishing their required concentrations.

But as important a nutrient as water is, it alone cannot keep us alive. In that regard, it is not a perfect nutrient. The best that we can say is that water, when untainted by chemicals, toxins, parasites, or pathogens, is the best liquid nutrient we can consume. Ultimately, water needs to work in concert with food to sustain us. Were we only to subsist on water, taking in no food whatsoever, we would live about a month or so and then die from starvation. If we introduced food to our water fast, effectively ending the fast, obviously, we'd live, even if the foods added were unhealthful foods in the form of cakes, hot dogs, burgers, chips, salty processed foods, and sugary cereals. How can this be when I've clearly and emphatically explained to you how harmful these foods are? I appear to be contradicting myself and seem to be saying that, then, there are no bad foods. That's not what I'm saying at all. I'll get back to this.

Plain broccoli is generally considered a healthful food. I don't think the vast majority of the population would find this to be a controversial statement, regardless of their personal feelings about broccoli. But if you were to eat nothing but healthful, plain broccoli, you would eventually die from any of a number of diseases brought about by malnutrition. If you were to eat nothing but apples, another food broadly viewed as healthful, you would die from a disease induced by malnutrition. Consumed exclusively, specific foods generally regarded as healthful are not perfect because while each food may contain nutrients similar to a different food, basically overlapping a nutrient (vitamin C is found in grapefruit, cauliflower, green bell peppers, spinach, and broccoli, for example) each individual food also contains its own particular set of nutrients. Unlike some creatures in the animal kingdom, humans did not evolve in such a specialized way so as to be able to eat only one thing to the basic exclusion of all others. We are not like giant pandas who, by and large, subsist only on bamboo as a food source. We require a variety of foods to provide us with all the nutrients needed in order for us to survive and thrive.

Think back to your history lessons about poorly nourished sailors afflicted with scurvy brought about by a lack of vitamin C. Consider the many poor and developing nations of today's world where people are suffering from pellagra, a disease caused by a deficiency in vitamin B3 (niacin). Vitamin A deficiency can cause blindness. A lack of fat is not a problem usually associated with the American diet, but most have heard about how some female athletes disrupt their hormonal systems by drastically lowering their body fat to unhealthy levels, to the point of causing a cessation of their menstrual cycles.

It's well known that a diet low in fiber is linked to colon cancer. From vitamins to protein and every essential nutrient in between, there exists a disease or affliction for every deficiency. Sometimes, nutrient inadequacy is caused by the body's inability to absorb a certain nutrient due to a genetic or medical problem, despite the fact that an individual may actually be ingesting foods containing the required nutrient.

Conversely, there exist medical conditions caused by consuming too much of a particular nutrient, as I pointed out a few paragraphs ago using water as the example. There is such a thing as vitamin toxicity, particularly among the fat-soluble vitamins A, D, E, and K, which the body stores in our fat and liver. The body utilizes and disposes of these vitamins at a much slower rate than the water-soluble vitamins, including vitamin C and the B complex vitamins, which need to be replaced on a more frequent basis. Taking too much of a water-soluble vitamin, especially in the form of supplements, usually results in, as the saying goes, "expensive urine" because the body will eliminate the excess. However, your health can be threatened by some water-soluble vitamins taken in doses regarded as toxic, such as vitamin B6 (pyridoxine), an excess of which can cause sensitivity to light, skin sores, and if megadoses are continued long enough, they can cause nerve damage. Unsafe doses of vitamin B3 (niacin) can result in skin flushing, nausea, diarrhea, and liver damage. Too much vitamin C (ascorbic acid) may induce symptoms such as diarrhea, vomiting, and headache.

As with vitamins, which in proper amounts are necessary to our well-being, so goes the story for minerals, chemical elements and metals in our diet. Some minerals are also characterized as chemical elements and metals. I won't get into a chemistry lesson here, so suffice to say that iron and copper are two which fall into this category. The human body requires both to carry out some of its normal functions, and these two are, among others, such as manganese, iodine, zinc, molybdenum, chromium, and selenium, considered essential to that end. The jury is still out on whether the controversial mineral fluorine is an essential mineral or one that causes more harm than good. All of the minerals mentioned in this paragraph are categorized as trace minerals because as much as the body needs them for good health, they are only required in minute amounts.

The other category of essential nutritional minerals is that category which contains the macro minerals. The body requires larger doses of these for it to function optimally than those required of trace minerals. Among the macro minerals are calcium, phosphorus, magnesium, potassium, sulfur, sodium, and chloride. Whether macro or trace, one thing that nutritional minerals have in common with vitamins is that too much or too little can harm us.

And, of course, there exist those vexing questions concerning the absolute certainty as to what amount and degree members of the family of minerals classified as heavy metals, including arsenic, mercury, lead, cadmium, aluminum, and uranium, present potential danger to human health. It's bad enough that these minerals occur naturally in the soil in some areas where our food crops are planted. However, it's an absolute travesty that they are present as a result of human activity. Humanity appears to be engaged in a drawn-out suicide by tainting the very resources— soil, water and air— that sustain our lives, the end result of usually placing profit before the health of the people.

It can be quite disheartening to be seriously committed to a healthful way of eating when you find out that the organic produce or plant-based, organic protein powder you purchased is not spared from the potentiality of being poisoned by toxic heavy metals. Even the organic label can't save us here.

To further muddy up the waters, there is the issue of certain nutrients and compounds blocking the absorption of other nutrients. Oxalic acid, found in green leafy vegetables, can attach itself to calcium and prevent its absorption. Phytic acid, found in whole grains, seeds, some nuts, and legumes, can diminish the amount of calcium and magnesium the body absorbs. Tannins in tea and coffee can decrease the absorption of iron. These and various other compounds are found in healthful, plant-based foods and are referred to as anti-nutrients. Anti-nutrients are a plant's natural defense against insects and bacteria. The effects of some anti-nutrients can be rendered harmless, limited or eradicated by soaking or boiling the food, such as in the case of dried beans and peas for example.

And what of essential nutrients disrupting one another? Most nutrients, such as vitamins and minerals, work with one another in numerous known combinations and in other ways which science has yet to discover. A couple of examples of partnerships among nutrients include vitamin D helping the body to absorb calcium and vitamin C assisting in the body's absorption of non-heme iron (the form of iron found in plant-based foods). Some minerals, regardless of the fact that they work together, actually compete for absorption. Such an example is the working relationship between zinc and copper.

I can easily understand how a person can become confused, frustrated, and downright angry by the concept of healthful eating. Some people contend that it makes no difference what one eats because there's something wrong, to one degree or another, with everything we eat. The argument has some merit.

Others, including many nutritionists, believe that no food is bad and that a well-balanced diet includes all things in—here comes that word again—moderation. I strongly disagree, and I'll refer to what I stated some paragraphs ago, where you might think I was contradicting myself by adding junk foods to a water fast to keep us alive. Yes, ceasing a water-only diet by consuming unhealthful cakes, hotdogs, burgers, chips, salty processed foods, and sugary cereals would save our lives from starvation in the short term. Most unhealthful foods, including fast foods, typical snack foods, common highly processed packaged foods, and junk food in general, contain at least a smattering of nutrients essential for sustaining life—at least enough to keep us alive for a while. In the long term, a steady diet of these types of foods would lead to a variety of easily preventable diseases in the best case scenario and a premature death in the worst case scenario.

The problem is that the downside of eating these unhealthful foods, by far, outweighs the upside of their consumption unless, of course, you are starving. The smidgen of nutritional value they contain is negated by the varying presence and combinations of high sodium, saturated fat, partially hydrogenated oils, sugar, artificial colors, and a hodgepodge of other man-made chemicals that no sane person would ever mention in the same breath as with real food.

Barring a food allergy, special need, medical condition, or being stranded on a desert island where I would eat boiled Spam to survive if nothing else were available, then, most certainly, a particular method of eating must be adhered to for optimum health. Eating unhealthful food in moderation or encouraging people to do so sends mixed messages and shows, by my way of thinking, a lack of commitment and a feckless character, producing an overabundance of excuses. It's a clear recipe for setting everyone up for failure. It's easy to be swept up by the hype employed by the food and beverage industries—the feelings of excitement, nostalgia, sexiness, trendiness, fun, tastiness, and general coolness elicited by their products—through slickly constructed advertising campaigns. All this while downplaying or ignoring the extremely negative health ramifications of their wares. At times, many even boast of the addition of a healthful ingredient in an effort to add health legitimacy to an otherwise unhealthful product. The food and beverage industries are in business to make money, not to look after your health; that's your job. They continue to misinform and manipulate the population into believing in the worthiness of their worthless products. People need to make informed choices about eating for health, not choices based on deception.

If you're overweight and out-of-shape and are content to spend most of your time burrowed into your couch cushions each day, wolfing down candy, chips, take-out, and gulping soda while watching daytime (or nighttime, for that matter) trash TV, great, at least you're content. It's not my job to brainwash you. I'm only here to present a different perspective. We can still be friends. But if you tell me that the chips are the low-salt variety, so they are better for your health, and the candy is the low-sugar version, and the soda is diet, then you, my friend, are an advertiser's dream come true. You are a happily manipulated result of great advertising and marketing strategy. There are many of you out there, and you have been, and continue to be, duped. They are telling you just what you want to hear.

When I considered the upsides and downsides of all the foods and beverages of which I'm familiar, a plant-based diet always came out on top. The positives of a plant-based diet far outweigh the negatives, and the negatives of any other way of eating, to my mind, far exceed any positive benefits they may impart. For example, deli meats may contain protein, but the sodium, fat, type of protein, and type of nitrites/nitrates they contain preclude me from including them in my diet. Low sugar and low sodium processed foods may be better than the originals, in all their sugary and salty glory, but better doesn't make something healthful. It's merely a statistical term. Soda is worthless garbage, and alcohol, despite the health claims, is a disinfectant not fit for human consumption. You can keep the vineyards and ludicrously expensive wines along with their fancy tastings. I'm not impressed.

I scoff at the notion that some consider me to be abnormal and extreme. Remember that in America, the vast majority of the population is overweight and in horrendous physical condition. Also, the bulk (pun intended) became this way as a result of their own choices. This is our normal. I want no part of that normal because it's killing us. If it's considered abnormal and extreme to avoid all the unreasonably inane things that so many people engage in, unnecessarily posing risks to their health, while exercising and eating the best food available to promote one's health, then yes, I'm abnormal, and I wouldn't have it any other way. The world is a strange place when you consider that those who are doing their best to harm themselves are encouraged, supported, and looked upon as normal, while those who take good care of their health are labeled as extremists.

Unless you've been living in a cave for the last 50 years, having had no contact with civilization, such as it is, the overwhelming majority of reasonably functioning adults on the planet are aware that added sugar and sodium, trans-fat, saturated fat, artificial colors, artificial preservatives, pesticides, fungicides, herbicides, white flour, white rice, white pasta, white bread, animal flesh, dairy, antibiotics, hormones, hydrogenated oils, HFCS, artificial sweeteners, alcohol, soda (diet or otherwise), deli meats and a slew of difficult to pronounce chemicals are having a negative impact on the health of humanity. This, actually, is an understatement. It's the catastrophe that virtually no one wants to address, except in a pandering manner, for fear of turning people off and angering large corporations producing edible and drinkable products that strongly contribute to preventable diseases and premature death. We have been set up to view ourselves as victims, thus avoiding responsibility for our actions.

As I stated earlier, but it bears repeating, eating even the foods that I've repudiated and foods infused with any of the questionable additives I've mentioned would keep you from starving. They contain nutrients your body requires in addition to things that your body does not require and will cause you harm. So, given a choice of irrefutably more healthful foods like fresh vegetables and fruits, whole grains, raw nuts, seeds, beans and legumes, even with their downside, the obvious choice is the plant-based diet. I don't believe in a middle ground here. You are either doing all you can to improve and maintain your health, or you're not. Eat the best foods you can. Don't eat bad food, not even in moderation. Consuming harmful foods and beverages in moderation is like hitting yourself in the head with a rock—but only occasionally.

We need to change the cultural way we think about certain things we moderately ingest, referring to them as treats and rewards. These treats and rewards, as they are tediously declared, have to be seen for the injurious substances they really are and recognized for the havoc they wreak on the human body. With the damage that these substandard foods inflict on the collective health of society, it should not matter how good they taste.

Many things we encounter in life feel good, look good, and taste good, but it doesn't necessarily follow that these things are, in fact, good for us at all. I have never had an interest in trying recreational drugs because their use is counter to everything in which I believe. However, it is my understanding that the first-ever line of cocaine, shot of heroin, or hit of crystal meth is supposed to deliver a tremendous high, resulting in the user feeling great, euphoric—better than anything ever experienced. You'd be an idiot to willfully engage in behaviors such as these.

You may be thinking that comparing the use of recreational drugs to the consumption of harmful foods is quite a stretch. You may be of the opinion that I'm conflating two very different social issues. I bring these two issues together because I believe that more people die in America, directly or indirectly, from their eating habits than from all illegal, recreational drugs combined. Recall that approximately 75% of America is overweight, but not even close to 75% of America is addicted to illegal, recreational drugs—not even remotely close. The problem here is that in a polite, conventional society, being overweight, despite being a well-known risk to health and life, is not illegal, not that I'm suggesting it should be.

No one need fear that such a law will come to pass to persecute the overweight as a result of their own asinine behaviors. The fact is that almost everyone in the country, including so many of our supposed leaders and other authoritative figures tasked with running the madness that is this show, are overweight, out-of-shape, and engage in a dizzying host of behaviors that negatively impact their very own health. This, while hypocritically paying nothing but lip service to the real idea of healthful living. In addition, they promote ridiculously tortured efforts, campaigns, and ideas that provide no more than the appearance of giving a damn about the health and well-being of the citizenry. Therefore, no need to worry; it's obvious why such legislation will never be delivered.

Meanwhile, the government has been waging the "war on drugs" for over a generation. As this war continues to be waged, a more insidious enemy persists in ravaging America, growing ever more powerful with each passing year and causing far greater casualties. Unfortunately, the reality is that, in a general sense, we don't really want to see or believe it. I have yet to hear of a war declaration on disease and death promoting shit food.

164

No, no food is perfect. Life isn't perfect; that's reality, and you either deal with it or psychologically crumble. Life is lived one decision at a time. Will I eat this or not? Will I exercise or not? Will I get enough sleep or not? Just about every daily decision we make impacts our physical and mental health in one way or another. A wrong decision can begin a domino effect of further wrong decisions. This can, in turn, initiate the building of a foundation of harmful habits. Sometimes, the damage is so great that it cannot be undone. You need to consider just how much your life is worth.

With food, as with life chiefly, the best course of action is to always place the odds in your favor. You do this by weighing the pros and cons of the food that is available to you. Always seek out the most healthful choice, even if the options all seem to be poor. I would advise you, if at all possible, to not place yourself in a position where all food options seem to be poor. If you are fortunate enough, and in this country most of us are, to be able to choose between a good (meaning far superior) food and an obviously bad (meaning far inferior) food, don't rationalize, simply choose the good food.

39

What To Eat And Drink
(Barring Allergies, Other Medical Conditions And Special Needs)

Fruits and Vegetables

If we lived in a flawless world where everything was transparent, and there weren't so many people motivated by money, stepping on others in an unapologetic effort to get this money, I would simply advise you to eat organic fruits and vegetables. The toxins used in conventional agriculture to protect crops from infestations of insects, fungi, and weeds and to produce higher crop yields may make your produce pretty, but they are not fit for human consumption nor that of any other living creature, no matter how enthusiastically they are greenwashed or healthwashed by those promoting them. Conventional farming threatens not only the health of the individual consumer but also the quality of groundwater and the ecosystem in general with its abundance of varied lifeforms.

From a health perspective and a "good of the people" point of view, the idea of organic agriculture is wonderful. It basically means that produce is grown without the addition of manmade chemicals, hormones, or drugs. No rationally thinking person wants to eat pesticides. Unfortunately, but typically, if there is a buck to be made somewhere, those blinded by greed will find a way to game the system by manipulating, obfuscating, making deals, compromising, rationalizing, endorsing, and finally spinning their tale to a public that is far too often impressionable and easily fooled. I like to keep things simple. It stands to reason that the more chemicals we are exposed to, the more we increase our odds of something going dreadfully wrong. In my simple world, organic agriculture would mean what it was originally intended to mean. It would mean that no manmade chemicals of any kind would be used in the growing, harvesting, or handling of organic produce, period. This is unambiguous and easily understood. However, the reality is that organic standards vary country by country and with so much produce being imported into the United States, because we can't live without summer fruit in the dead of winter, this creates a problem.

To further confuse the organic issue, the authorities in charge of organic standards make exceptions, as they deem necessary, for certain synthetic substances. Also, consumers need to be aware that not all organic labels on multi-ingredient foods are identical. There's a difference between 100% Organic (this speaks for itself), Organic (95% of the ingredients certified organic by USDA), Made With Organic (must contain at least 70% organic ingredients), and Organic

Ingredients (less than 70% of the ingredients are certified organic). It's important to know this so you can better make an informed decision regarding what you choose to eat and have it be within your comfort zone. Pay attention when shopping for food. Don't be fooled by food packaging boasting a label with the word "Organic." Ask yourself if the product is 100% organic, 95% organic, made of at least 70% organic ingredients, or contains less than 70% organic ingredients.

I didn't get to this point in my life by having blind faith, least of all when it comes to government officials and policymakers. I believe a good dose of healthy doubt is in order when it comes to these people. Most individuals have an agenda; those in charge are no different. I'm not implying that there exists a coordinated government conspiracy to screw the public, only that there are too many in public service who cherish their positions of power and the prospect of adding to their net worth far more than they embrace their roles as the implementers of good public policies and as guardians of those policies. On the other hand, a bit of faith is not always a bad thing. As such, and in line with my comfort level, when the USDA (United States Department of Agriculture) certifies a food with one of its "Organic" labels, I accept it for what it is, albeit with a robust but un-paralyzing dose of skepticism. I'm making an educated gamble here. I choose to believe that they're "probably" on the level, but in the survival center of my mind I'm always thinking that nothing would surprise me.

I believe that organic farming is best overall for the health and well-being of the population, and I contend that it serves the environment as well. As such, I consume organic produce, but not if the food in question has a thick skin, since I'm not going to eat it. I don't overburden myself with personal health concerns over the organic nature, or lack thereof, of fruits and vegetables such as oranges, grapefruits, bananas, melons, avocados, jicama and nuts, to name but a few. Some may criticize me by pointing out that my selective eating of organic food is not one hundred percent in the best interests of the earth. They would be correct in this observation. I offer no apology for this seemingly glaring oversight of my commitment to all things health. I will only offer, by way of explanation, that my health and welfare comes first, an insignificant issue in the grand scheme of the universe, to be sure, but immensely important to me. I'll concern myself with the grand mission of healing the earth and its environment with the same diligence and fervor reserved for my wellness when I and my little life bubble are completely healed, and the task of fixing the earth doesn't appear to me as just shoveling crap against the tide. I'm just trying to get through each day here.

Organic food is usually more expensive than regular pesticide-laden food. If you can't afford organic produce, buy the regular variety and make sure to wash it under cool, running water. I suggest washing all produce under cool, running water, whether it's the regular kind or the organic variety, just to be on the safe side. Remember to place the odds in your favor to maximize your chances of survivability. Even produce encased in skin that you may want to peel off or slice through should be washed first. Running a knife or other utensil through this skin may force pesticides and other toxins into the edible flesh of that fruit or vegetable.

Don't kill or mitigate the inherent nutritional value of untainted produce, whether fresh, frozen, or packaged, by adding any unsavory additives, such as salt, sugar, hydrogenated oils, or processed salad dressings. Fruits can be eaten raw out of hand, in salads, in smoothies and in hot or cold healthful, whole-grain cereals. They can also be cooked in a variety of ways and can be combined with other wholesome ingredients to make healthfully delicious chutneys.

Many vegetables can also be eaten raw out of hand, in salads, mixed with various whole grains, or sautéed with garlic and other spices to make healthful and very tasty vegetable stews. Vegetables can also be combined with fruits to make smoothies, but don't limit yourself to the marriage of vegetables and fruits in smoothies alone. Use your imagination, be creative, and experiment because the possibilities are almost endless. Discover the combinations and recipes that most suit your palate. Just in case you're thinking about it, the answer is no; broccoli drowning under an ocean of cheese sauce is absolutely not on my list of recommended ways to eat vegetables.

Beans and Legumes

Beans and legumes are excellent sources of protein and fiber. They are an excellent addition to any whole-grain dish. If you are pressed for time and are reluctant to soak and properly cook the dry variety, you can use the canned, packaged, or Tetra-Pak varieties. Beware, however, that a pitfall of using pre-cooked beans off the grocery store shelf, no matter how they're packaged, is that they usually contain added salt. Lower salt-added options are making some inroads into communities where consumers demand them. I view these options as weak and insignificant efforts to bring the best food to the masses. Some stores grudgingly stock a few no-salt-added varieties for the most astute shoppers. The unsalted versions are the most difficult to find because, unfortunately, the demand simply isn't there. The best of these types of products contain beans and water, nothing else. For your best health, this is what you should buy if you don't feel up to dealing with dry beans, not that doing so is really such a big deal.

If circumstances dictate and you are forced to use the regular, salted type or the low-sodium kind of beans or legumes, when opening the package, dump them into a colander and rinse them thoroughly under cool, running water to remove as much salt as possible. This is a good example of choosing a superior food that has been rendered less than superior by the addition of an undesirable ingredient, namely, salt, in this instance. We can easily ascertain the upside as well as the downside. This is an illustration of how we rectify, as best we can, the downside. In a better and smarter world, all pre-cooked and packaged beans and legumes would be unsalted, rendering this method of improving or "fixing" our food unnecessary. Unfavorably, this is not a better world, nor by most appearances, do large numbers of us seem to be getting smarter, so the logical among us must take matters into our own hands.

As a side note, another way to get beans into your diet is to occasionally mix it up by eating pasta made from 100% bean or lentil flour. Also, when baking, combine whole-wheat flour with bean flour. There are quite a few varieties available, including black bean and garbanzo bean.

Nuts, Drupes, and Seeds

Seeds—sunflower, pumpkin, poppy, sesame, and nuts and drupes—almonds, peanuts (which are not really nuts but legumes), Brazil nuts, pine nuts, walnuts, chestnuts, pecans, pistachios, filberts (also known as hazelnuts), cashews and others, are packed with nutrition. They are good sources of protein, healthful fat, fiber, vitamins, and minerals. Eat them raw or dry roasted, not salted, glazed, or with other additives. Once salt, sugar, or oil are added to them, a good food is reduced to a junk food. Nuts, drupaceous nuts, and seeds can be sprinkled on fresh fruit, hot or cold whole-grain cereal, and included in whole-grain pancakes, waffles, muffins, cakes, cookies, and pies (yes, the healthful versions you make in your own kitchen). They can be added to whole-grain dishes such as pasta, millet, barley, oatmeal, quinoa, teff, farro, and others in a similar fashion as beans and legumes are added. They're great in salads. Flax seeds, especially when ground, are also a healthful addition to your diet. They have slowly but steadily been gaining a foothold on some grocery store shelves and are becoming more mainstream. Besides contributing the dietarily essential nutrients that seeds are known for—protein, fiber, vitamins, and minerals—flax seeds add all-important omega-3 fatty acids to the diet.

Nut and seed butters and the like are, generally speaking, healthful and nutritious foods. They are high in protein, contain fiber and some healthful fats. The problem with healthful nut butters is trying to find them because most mainstream brands contain other ingredients besides nuts. If you look at the ingredients label on a jar of peanut butter, for example, the only ingredient you will see on the better brands is peanuts. That's it, nothing else. If you take a jar of peanut butter off the grocery store shelf and see that it contains anything other than peanuts, even if it's only salt, then that healthful product has been degraded. Adding salt, sugar, sweeteners (natural or not), hydrogenated oils, purportedly healthful substances, or anything for that matter, does not improve the healthfulness of peanut butter or any nut/seed butter. It makes no difference what spin the manufacturers of additive-containing, mainstream nut butters put on their products; their nut butters are healthfully inferior to those containing only nuts. Keep it simple. Least I forget, lose the typical jellies and jams that most people combine with nut/seed butters unless you're using those that are only sweetened with fruit juice. Plain apple butter is another good choice. Nut/seed butters with sliced fresh fruit is yet another option. And, as with beans, another alternative for adding the benefits of nuts to your diet is to use flour made from 100% ground-up nuts, such as hazelnuts or almonds, in combination with whole-wheat flour when you bake.

Grains In General

When it comes to eating grains, only whole grains are acceptable. Processed grains—those which are not 100% whole—have been stripped of essential nutrients, especially fiber, and are nutritionally inferior to whole grains. There are many varieties of whole grains available, including whole-wheat bread (be mindful with this one because most commercially available bread, even those boasting a whole-wheat or whole-grain label, are not worth eating due to the inclusion of unacceptable ingredients), cereals and pastas, amaranth, quinoa, teff, millet, farro, spelt, oatmeal, barley, freekeh, fonio, buckwheat, kamut, sorghum and kaniwa. When baking, making pancakes, waffles, or whatever your cooking needs, use only 100% whole-grain flour such as whole-wheat, rye, buckwheat, and whole-oat flour. For additional fiber, vitamins, and minerals, include wheat germ, unprocessed oat or wheat bran, or ground psyllium husks in your baking, cooking, salads, cereals, smoothies, and whichever other culinary ideas come to mind. Whole grains are nutrient-rich and good-for-you carbohydrates. The carbohydrates to stay away from are those which are processed. If you have any white flour lying around, the only thing that's good for, as I stated pages ago, is when you're involved in an art project which requires the making of papier-mâché.

Brewer's Yeast and Nutritional Yeast

Brewer's yeast and nutritional yeast can be added to baked goods, pancakes, waffles, cereals, and smoothies. Nutritional yeast can also be sprinkled on whole-grain dishes such as pasta, for example, instead of grated cheese. It has a nice, sharp, nutty flavor reminiscent of a pungent cheese. Once you become accustomed to it, you'll crave it on all the dishes where you would have previously used grated cheese. Brewer's yeast has a slightly more bitter but certainly not unpleasant flavor. Both nutritional yeast and brewer's yeast are good sources of protein, vitamins, and minerals.

Cereal

As I mentioned in my general statements concerning grains, obviously, the same holds true for cereal. Cereal, being made from grains, should only be eaten in the 100% whole-grain version. This is the most healthful type, whether hot or cold. Oatmeal, puffed whole oats, puffed whole wheat, amaranth, whole-kamut puffs, whole-corn puffs, shredded whole wheat, and puffed whole millet are a few examples. Make sure they contain absolutely no added sweeteners, sodium, milk chocolate, marshmallows, or any of the other crap that mainstream cereal manufacturers add to their products to tempt children and childlike adults.

Be vigilant as to the presence of butylated hydroxytoluene (BHT), a preservative and suspected carcinogen. If your cereal is preserved with anything, be sure that it is vitamin E (mixed tocopherols) only. Other than the possibility of this vitamin E preservative, there should be nothing other than whole grain, a combination of whole grains, or dry roasted/raw seeds and nuts. Add your own fresh, frozen, or dry fruit if you desire to sweeten it. If your supermarket has no healthful cereals to choose from and you must base your choice on the lesser of evils, remember that all mainstream cereals contain, at the very least, added salt and sugar in varying amounts. Pick the cereal with the least added salt and sugar.

Some people think that Cheerios are a healthful cereal. Compared to Lucky Charms, which contain, of all things, marshmallow bits, among other unacceptable ingredients, I suppose one could reasonably argue that they are. In reality, Cheerios also contain added salt and sugar. However, if it were a choice between Cheerios and Lucky Charms, I'd reluctantly choose Cheerios. To be clear, I need to stress that all foods, meals, snacks, beverages, anything you eat should be the most healthful available. Cheerios could fall into that category if nothing better is available and only when compared to an even worse choice, but make no mistake, in the grand scheme of things Cheerios do not qualify as one of the healthful cereals.

Sweeteners

Sweeteners used for baking and other cooking needs should be limited to a minimal amount of fruit juice, raw honey, 100% maple syrup, or blackstrap molasses. They contain vitamins and minerals and are better than their "light" or "diet" versions, which are basically laboratory fabrications. Use these sweeteners sparingly, even though they are better alternatives than processed sugars. You want to allow your taste buds to rebound from years of abuse, which have denied you the ability to actually taste the food. In due time, a sparse amount of these recommended sweeteners will be all you need as you, once again or perhaps for the first time, experience enjoying the flavor of healthful food while simultaneously indulging your sweet tooth. Unsweetened baby food is also a good choice as a sweetener, such as bananas, pears or apples. You can also mash your own fresh fruit.

Dried Fruit

There is a wide variety of dried fruit on the market today, but it is not all created equally. Raisins, prunes, apples, figs, dates, apricots, currents, golden berries, cranberries, and more can be found in most decent grocery stores. They can all be a positive addition to your diet. Trying to find dried fruit without added sugar, artificial sweeteners, or even without the acceptable sweeteners I mentioned in the "Sweeteners" section is the challenge. Dried fruit is sweet enough on its own due to the dehydration process, causing the natural sugars in the fruit to become very concentrated and requires no further sweetening. Adding sweeteners simply adds unnecessary calories. Undaunted, food manufacturers persist in piling on more sugar to an already sweet product. They're not doing you any favors.

Pineapple, mango, papaya, blueberries, cranberries and bananas are some of the most difficult varieties of dried fruit to find in their unsweetened versions. This problem is often compounded by the addition of not only sweeteners but vegetable oil as well. This holds true whether you are seeking them out in mainstream supermarkets or in the trendy, allegedly healthful shopping emporiums. They're not impossible to find, just difficult. Look at an ordinary container of raisins. Why is oil an additive?! Don't give up because the unsweetened/oil-free varieties of dried fruit do exist.

Dried fruit can be added to salad, cereal, baked goods, or eaten right out of the package. It can be mixed with raw or dry roasted nuts and seeds to make your own wholesome trail mix right at home. Make sure you are not allergic to the preservative sulfur dioxide found in many dried fruits. Better yet, hold out until you locate dried fruit without this or any other chemical preservative. Just as dried fruit without added sweeteners and oils can be found, it is possible to find it without chemical preservatives. I can't remind you enough to read the labels.

Canned Fruit

Canned fruit can also be a healthful addition to your dietary habits. However, as I have already illustrated, no food is perfect. A couple of downsides of canned fruit is that it is most often found in heavy or light syrup packed in BPA (bisphenol A) lined cans. BPA is an industrial chemical used in the manufacture of certain plastics. It is a known endocrine disruptor and can potentially cause other health problems.

Canned fruit swimming in heavy syrup is an unnecessary redundancy. Food producers are guilty once again of attempting to suffocate us under an avalanche of sugar. This is another example of adding something sweet to something that is already naturally sweet providing you with more useless, empty calories. When choosing canned fruit, purchase only those that are packed in either 100% fruit juice or, an even better choice are, those packed in water. If any other sweeteners or additives are included, place the can back on the shelf.

Oil, Butter, and The Like

Extra virgin olive oil is my oil of choice. However, I only use it on extremely rare occasions, perhaps 2 or 3 times per year, despite the rave reviews concerning the Mediterranean Diet. A serving size consists of 1 tablespoon (about 15 ml) and contains about 120 calories, all of them fat calories. The total fat included in one serving is 14 g, 2 g of which is saturated fat, 1.5 g of polyunsaturated fat, and 10 g of monounsaturated fat. As you can see, most of the fat in olive oil is currently considered to be good fat.

Some believe other oils provide health benefits, too, such as peanut oil, coconut oil, avocado oil, and canola oil. You'll encounter quite a bit of controversy and disagreement when it comes to the purported health advantages of different oils. They are definitely not the same. Do some research instead of falling for the hype. Personally, I have virtually eliminated all oils from my diet due to the damage they may cause to the epithelial cells which line our blood vessels.

As far as butter is concerned, I never use it, not only because it's an animal derivative, but due to the high percentage of saturated fat it contains. Margarine is absolutely out of the question. It is nothing more than partially hydrogenated oil, which contains trans-fat. This will clog your arteries with wax-like cholesterol, setting you up nicely for a potential heart attack or stroke. You can keep all those other fake butter/margarine spreads that are supposedly so heart-healthy. As far as I'm concerned, the positive health proclamations delivered in the ads far exceed the reality.

Beverages

Water, by far, should be the beverage of choice. I believe most city water supplies in America to be relatively safe but I also believe in overkill when it comes to my health. One need look no further than Flint, Michigan, and Newark, New Jersey, to find examples where city water supply systems tragically failed the citizenry. If you can afford it, install a reverse osmosis or other water filtration system in your home. This is important even if you live in a rural area where your drinking water is sourced from a well. Much of the water in rural aquifers, in parts of the country, traditionally and mythologically associated with clean, fresh, wholesome, natural living, is being poisoned due to toxins being introduced into groundwater by polluters from various industries. These industries include but are not limited to, coal-fired power plants, mining, hydraulic fracturing or fracking, and numerous manufacturers that illegally dump a witch's brew of poisons onto our land and into our waters. While these industries provide numerous jobs and economic growth, their waste disposal methods are irresponsible.

I prefer to exercise on an empty stomach, so to speak. After a good night's sleep, I drink about 2 ounces of 100% fruit juice, followed by at least 8 ounces of water. Then I work out. After a full night of sleep and not eating anything for about eight hours or so (unless you're guilty of making nocturnal refrigerator raids), your blood sugar is relatively low. The juice "breaks the fast," which, by the way, is the genesis of the word breakfast and boosts my blood sugar just enough so that I can function in the gym.

The more pulp juice contains, the better it is for you. Notice that I mentioned 100% fruit juice, not juice drink. Juice drinks are nothing more than soft drinks disguised as something wholesome. They contain some actual juice but are diluted with water and contain sweeteners, including HFCS, and usually, other less-than-ideal ingredients. However, don't be seduced into the belief that a large 8-ounce glass of real fruit juice is necessarily in your best interest. Many actual fruit juices contain as much sugar as soda.

Have you ever thought about how "soft drinks" is such a benign-sounding moniker? They can't possibly cause any harm because, after all, they're soft, unlike booze, which is hard. Humans are so easily manipulated by nice-sounding words. The reality is that soda, whether diet or regular, sports drinks, energy drinks, sweetened teas, and all the rest of these mass-marketed potions are simply liquid junk food. Diet soda, in particular, is problematic due to the general belief that it is a healthful alternative to regular soda because it is sugar-free. Lost in this belief is the fact that the artificial sweeteners and chemicals used in the manufacture of diet soda contribute their own array of potential health problems. These may include but are not limited to heart disease, diabetes, and obesity.

The majority of humanity is mentally weak and undisciplined. A small example of this weakness is exposed whenever someone says, "I can't get through the day without my coffee." Coffee has become yet another crutch that humans use to cope. As if the stimulating effects of caffeine on our hearts were not bad enough, coffee, once a simple beverage, has, in many instances, become a dessert when you consider the designer nature of what it has morphed into. Coffee is a multi-billion dollar-per-year enterprise fronted by trendy coffee shops that have coffee menus. Gone are the days of plain black coffee, coffee with a bit of milk, and "How many sugars?" Not that I'm glorifying that nonsense. My point is that the consumption of coffee has reached new levels of ridiculousness. These shops whip up many coffee confections with as many calories and heart stopping ingredients as a decadent sweet.

Since I mentioned coffee being a crutch which so many rely on, is there any bigger crutch than alcohol? Alcohol is the legal drug of the masses. It has far more downsides than upsides, despite the fact that researchers feverishly seek to discover any positive news about a substance that has caused untold misery throughout human existence. Nevertheless, alcohol has been promoted to the point where it is linked to so many warm and fuzzy, positive images. Think about the depictions you've seen of friends sharing beers while watching a sporting event, all manner of celebrations where the thought of not drinking would be outrageous, alcoholic beverages linked to fun, friends, family, manliness, sophistication, coolness, chicness, trendiness and traditions, which by the way, are not necessarily a good thing. An entire segment of the tourist industry is devoted to wineries and vineyards with particular emphasis in the United States on Napa Valley, California.

People seeking to become wine and wine service experts take accredited courses to become sommeliers. There even exists a ranking system among sommeliers depending on their level of education and knowledge. There are other courses available for individuals who are not interested in the service aspect of alcohol but wish to acquire tasting skills, a knowledge of a beverage's origin, and all things pertaining to alcohol. Then they can become wine snobs or snobs of whatever their hootch of choice is and will be able to brag about spending hundreds, thousands, or yes, as much as millions of dollars per bottle. Look it up. Sheer idiocy pretending to be high-class.

This, to me, is elitist bullshit at its best. A knowledge of alcohol? The fruity aromas, tartness, color, acidity, undertones of this or that, sweetness, body, complex textures, bouquet, who cares? In the grand scheme of things, it's one of the least important things a person can know. The only thing you need to know about alcohol is the harm it does to your body. It makes no difference what it costs per bottle. It doesn't matter that some make claims as to the heart health benefits alcohol is supposed to possess. No doctor in his or her right mind is going to suggest you begin imbibing to improve your heart health if you are a nondrinker to begin with. This doesn't sound like a rousing vote of confidence for the medicinal attributes of alcohol. You want heart health? Put down the drink, lose weight, eat properly, and do some vigorous cardio.

As far as milk is concerned, cow milk is for baby cows, goat milk is for baby goats, camel milk is for baby camels, yak milk is for baby yaks...well, I'm sure you get my point. Therefore, human milk is for baby humans. If you have a need to use a milk substitute, be sure to check the contents of your almond, cashew, oat, hemp, soy and the numerous other non-dairy alternatives available. Some contain oil, are high in sodium and contain undesirable ingredients such as carrageenan, which is a highly controversial food additive.

Animal Flesh

The consumption of animal flesh is generally unnecessary, not even the flesh of fish. I haven't included any creature from the animal kingdom in my diet in over twenty years. I have remained alive and in good health. As a matter of fact, to this point, I continue to be one of the healthiest and most fit, average persons I know.

Most animals raised and sold for food are pumped full of drugs in an effort to make them grow bigger in the shortest amount of time possible. These chemicals are also administered to fight off the diseases these animals inevitably fall victim to. The maladies which they contract are due, in part, to the horrendous circumstances in which they are kept. Filth and crowded conditions predominate. Their illnesses are exacerbated as a result of the diets forced upon them in an all-out effort by producers to maximize animal growth.

Some people argue that eating organically raised animals is a better option, not only for the humans consuming their flesh but for the animals themselves. The thought of organically raised, chemical-free animals being fed a wholesome diet, cavorting blissfully, free-range style, with members of their own species, prior to being "humanely executed, eviscerated, and butchered" has much public appeal. Lost in all the outpouring and support for animal sensibilities is the fact that despite being permitted what their human overlords consider a good life and death, animals still contain artery-clogging saturated fat and cholesterol. There is also the question of whether eating animal protein itself, regardless of saturated fat and cholesterol, is as healthful as humans have been spoon-fed to believe. I reject the overused marketing ploy encouraging us to eat "lean animal protein."

As for those on the seafood bandwagon, besides the fact that we need not eat these creatures, I believe they contain far too many toxins to even consider. Humans have only themselves to blame for this atrocity. Thanks to money trumping all else, many businesses and industries have regularly used Earth's watery environs as a giant sewer system for dumping deadly, destructive substances. As a result of this shortsighted, misguided, greedy, and stupid behavior, animals living in these toxified waters absorb the poisons, making them unfit and unsafe for consumption. Despite the authoritative guidelines regularly issued by the "experts" instructing me as to what constitutes a generally safe amount of poison to ingest, I remain disinterested in such opinions and far more interested in their motivation for those opinions. I prefer to not ingest any amount of poison if I can help it, but hey, that's me. Do as you wish. I'll remain steadfast in my nutritional practices—so far, so good.

In fantasy land, if you were able to prove to me that a particular animal or way of raising animals enabled them to be an almost perfect food source, with no negative health ramifications after eating them, we would arrive at the ultimate argument of ethics. The more we study animals, the more we learn about their capacity to experience fear, pain, loneliness, and suffering. This holds true for all animals despite the labels and categories humans impose upon them. Animals, whether domesticated, wild, raised for food or to decorate ourselves with their body parts or confined to laboratory cages until it becomes their turn to be dissected and experimented on, know agony.

I am not an animal lover in the traditional sense of the phrase. I don't keep companion animals. Many people keep animals because they just want to, not out of need. Pets, as they are more commonly referred to, are generally a pain in the ass. They cost you money, take up your time due to their needs and care, limit where you can go and what you can do, must be disciplined, and need to be raised as children do. Personally, I don't have the time or inclination. If they work for you, great.

I think the idea of people and animals working together is a good one. Fields such as search and rescue, law enforcement, the military, and assisting the physically and mentally challenged serve as a better fate for animals than eating them. Human behaviors such as keeping animals in zoos or exploiting them for our entertainment, particularly our gambling entertainment, don't strike me as examples of human compassion. They speak more of human arrogance. We decide which non-human living creatures will grace our dinner tables and our bodies, which ones will perform tricks for us, the ones we can subject to scientific studies, those which are permitted to live in our homes, those worthy enough to work alongside us and the ones we will simply stuff and mount as a display of our power and dominance over every living thing on earth.

I do not hunt. However, this is not the result of a freakish affinity for the beasts of the wild. I live in a rural part of the country that is also home to wild animals, which could conceivably cause me harm. I spend a good amount of time in the woods and enjoy observing nature, including the animals in their habitat. I would have no problem defending myself from an animal attack and killing the animal to save myself. Fortunately, this has never come to pass. I like to think that the animals and I have an unspoken understanding; I let them be if they let me be. The truth of the matter is that I have no desire or need to kill anything unless it poses a threat to me or a loved one. I think that killing animals is misguided and killing in general is a bad idea. That said, if you want to push me on the subject, it's possible that far more humans than animals need to be killed to make the planet a safer and better place. Unfortunately, unless the killing of an evil and despicable human is sanctioned by an all-knowing governing body, this action is against the law.

From the perspective of health, as it's impacted by nutrition, I am not only surviving but thriving. Why would I then cause the suffering of another creature, even though it's not of my species, by killing and eating it? I can only shake my head at so many of the self-proclaimed animal lovers. These are the very same people who may own a dog, a cat, and two canaries. They profess their love for and devotion to animals while ignoring the fact that they've devoured a sausage and pepperoni, personal pizza for lunch, and are in the midst of roasting a chicken for dinner. Maybe tomorrow they'll go to the circus to be entertained by animals who perform tricks for their pleasure. If the weather is chilly or they wish to appear stylish, they'll wear the fur or leather formerly worn by their original owners prior to their having been executed and skinned, all in the name of vanity. These people should be more specific when they haughtily and wrongfully claim to be animal lovers. What they actually mean is that they love to possess certain species of animals as pets, consider others only for their frivolous entertainment value, designate others as nothing more than providers of clothing, and find other animals so flavorful that they can't stop themselves from eating them. Animal lovers, indeed.

If these self-proclaimed animal lovers love animals as much as they allege, why do they demean, wear, and eat them? I suppose human entertainment, fashion, and taste buds take precedence over love every time. Human arrogance and stupidity know no bounds. I sometimes wonder what humans would think if a far superior alien race, which isn't saying a lot, considering the state of the world with humanity at the helm, invaded and took control of Earth. What if these advanced beings saw fit to raise humans in laboratories and perform scientific experiments on us to benefit their species? What if they found us to be a pleasurable diversion from their boring, alien lives because we were trained to entertain them with tricks, as we do to orcas, dolphins, elephants, and a host of other creatures? What if they were degenerate gamblers and concocted athletic competitions pitting humans against one another so that they could wager on the outcome? Oh, that's right, we already do that to ourselves. What if they were sportsmen, as human hunters are referred to, and they hunted us for recreation, to cull our growing herd, or because alien fashion and style demanded the wearing of human skin and other body parts? What if the greedier among the aliens kept us in filthy, overcrowded pens, pumped us full of drugs to make us meatier and grow faster, all in the name of profit, and sold us as food because of the aliens' insatiable appetite for, what they considered, our tasty flesh? Would we feel any better about our plight as being the main course at Alien Thanksgiving, if we were raised by the more considerate alien organic human farmers? After all, as free-range, grass-fed humans, we'd have a wonderful existence, right? Perhaps this idea would make the benevolent among our new masters feel as good about themselves as we humans do when we make, as we see it, compassionate life-and-death decisions concerning Earth's "lesser" inhabitants.

40

Defining Good Health

Some time ago, I recall hearing on the radio a report about a survey revealing that 80% of Americans deemed themselves to be healthy. I was simultaneously fascinated and bemused upon hearing this considering that at the time, approximately 70% of Americans were overweight to one degree or another. I don't believe it's a stretch to state that many of America's inhabitants, if not the planet's, are a bit aware of at least some of the horrible medical conditions and diseases caused by being overweight. When you factor in the roughly 30 million diagnosed diabetics and nearly 3 times that number of people with pre-diabetes, that about half of all American adults have hypertension (high blood pressure), the more than 100 million people 20 years of age and older who have high cholesterol and just for good measure, tack on that nearly half of all adults in the U.S.A. have some form of cardiovascular disease, the numbers of this survey would have appeared laughable, were they not dangerously lulling a deluded population into comfortable denial.

The numbers simply didn't add up then and still don't. At this point, does anyone need to explain to the masses that being overweight usually causes or exacerbates what are mostly preventable illnesses? This drum has been beating for decades. America is a very sick and physically unfit nation and becoming more so with each passing day. Unfortunately, people will believe as they wish. What most of this country believes to be true and what the truth actually is are diametrically opposed. The former, most Americans consider themselves healthy, is wishful thinking, while the latter, most Americans are a hot mess, is certain.

Tune in to the media of your choice, and on an almost daily basis, the fact that we are fat, preventably sick, and physically unfit is emphasized relentlessly. On the other hand, but almost in the same breath, these same media outlets encourage us to consume more corn chips, drink more beer (responsibly, of course), and eat more fast food. This, coupled with pushing feckless ideas on what constitutes proper exercise, usually highlighting minimal amounts of time and barely breaking a sweat, is a recipe for the ever-worsening health crisis in which we find ourselves. Sadly, there is no end in sight because too many people refuse to see reality.

We persist in our hopeless attempts to lose weight and to become fit while neglecting to change enough of our suicidal habits to really make a difference. If you are honest for a moment, you'll plainly see that this line of thinking is failing on an epic scale. In this way, we resign ourselves to the notion that it's okay to live with diabetes, elevated cholesterol, high blood pressure, and heart disease because the truth is that, for the most part, we keep eating and drinking the same rubbish that we've always been eating and drinking. We are told that it's fine to continue with these poor habits that usually cause or worsen these deadly afflictions, but as long as we manage them with drugs from the ever-so-concerned-for-our-health pharmaceutical industry, we can rejoice. Just listen to their asinine jingles on any media. In fact, some become mini-musical productions that celebrate living joyfully with your disease. Although the potential side-effects are always mentioned, they lose their impact because of the up-beat presentation. The wasteland that is daytime network TV is replete with these commercials. A wonderful example is the one for Jardiance, an antidiabetic medication for people with type 2 diabetes, marketed by Boehringer Ingelheim and Eli Lilly and Company. Apparently, everyone in this commercial is living blissfully with their type 2 diabetes because they haven't suffered one of the potential side-effects, which is a life-threatening infection of the anus and genitals. If there's a Broadway in hell, this "musical" wins multiple Tony Awards.

If you go out in public, there's about a 75% chance you'll be looking at an overweight, out-of-shape person. Overweight has become the new normal. Many in our culture embrace this, focusing on the positive aspect of acceptance while completely ignoring the devastating health consequences of being overweight. I'm not talking about shaming people. I'm talking about telling the full story. Acceptance and inclusivity are wonderful, but not at the expense of destroying one's health or the health of future generations. There is no magic bullet, not even moderation. There are only behavioral changes, and yes, some require a bit of work. You shouldn't expect a good health outcome if you're taking actions that subvert this goal. You can't have it both ways—but we sure as hell are trying to and failing miserably in the process.

People buy into these twisted lines of truth because they're being told exactly what they want to hear. Full-grown, functioning adults are "drinking the Kool-Aid" being served up by a culture that is more concerned with soft, gentle, inoffensive words than with words such as responsibility, consequences, accountability, and harsh reality. The fact is, odds are if you live a certain way, you're going to get sick and die sooner than if you were to live another way. It's that simple. Disease or health. Life or death. The "choice," another important word, is yours. The prudent will learn all they can about health and life-promoting behaviors and put this knowledge into practice, increasing their chances of a long, healthy existence. The imprudent will be left weeping and bemoaning what they unrealistically believe to be their bad luck.

In my estimation, good health is the general nonexistence of disease, chronic medical condition or acute medical condition in an individual. Living with self-induced sickness by keeping it at bay through the use of multiple pharmaceuticals is not good health. That's like sticking another finger into yet another hole in a failing dike ready to burst and announcing that the dike is structurally sound. Good health and fitness go hand in hand. One could be disease-free but unable to climb a flight of stairs without becoming winded. In the past, if you spoke with many adults, they would affirm that they were living with at least one of the variety of potentially dangerous, usually self-inflicted medical conditions which I've mentioned numerous times. Today, young people suffer the same fate. No intelligent person would include any of these particular conditions as a necessary component of a "good health list."

Most people, healthy or not, at one time or another, experience one or a combination of the following: allergies, high blood pressure, elevated cholesterol, diabetes, insomnia, upper respiratory infections, headaches, irritable bowel syndrome, diarrhea, constipation, sinus issues, fungal infections, gas and bloating, acid reflux, vision problems, hearing impairment, dry or oily skin and hair, arthritis, bunions, corns, anxiety, chronic fatigue, halitosis, gum disease, tooth decay, brittle nails, acne, balance issues and vertigo, back pain, and ear infections, to name but a few of the maladies that afflict humanity. Obviously, some of these conditions are far more serious than others.

When healthy, fit people get sick, perhaps coming down with one of the aforementioned, less lethal conditions, they take the required medication, follow the correct protocols, and are usually back to normal in an acceptable period of time. This is a far cry from those people who have caused their own dangerous and unnecessary illnesses, such as heart disease, diabetes, hypertension, and elevated cholesterol, which are attributable almost exclusively to an existence of self-abuse. Everybody gets something, but unhealthy and unfit people are more prone to get the more life-threatening conditions and illnesses more often. This necessitates the "management" of these illnesses through drugs, or the results could be dire. People managing these suicidal diseases are not healthy, regardless of what they believe or what any survey reveals. They are only fooling themselves and merely marking time. Changing their eating habits combined with real exercise could, in most cases, reverse or eliminate these diseases. These folks could actually become healthy if they took the proper corrective actions. Just as I don't believe in the existence of perfect diets or perfect exercises, I don't believe in the existence of perfect health. Perfection is unachievable. There is only one's best health. This is entirely achievable if we choose to challenge ourselves by setting the bar high enough and working to see how close we come.

Catching the common cold, typical indigestion, a bout of diarrhea, and the familiar aches and pains caused by living, unlike some of the medical conditions known to kill the most Americans, such as heart disease, stroke, cancer, lung disease, Alzheimer's and diabetes, are predominately of little concern. However, knowing your body and self-monitoring is always a good idea. Like most people, if you periodically suffer from one or more of these non-life-threatening conditions but consider yourself healthy, you may be mistaken. The condition might be a symptom of an underlying, far more serious factor. Or, it could be nothing serious at all. If you are suspicious or apprehensive about a health concern that doesn't look or feel like what you're familiar with, consult with a trusted healthcare provider.

If you are living your best healthful life—eating properly, exercising, and doing all the other things within your power to promote your well-being—but you happen to become ill with something beyond your control, take some solace in the fact that you are indeed doing what you possibly can to remain healthy for as long as you can. Don't worry about it; it's wasted emotion. Simply keep doing what you're doing and move on. Life happens to everyone, no matter how we live. The best we can do is to minimize the amount of unpleasantness that befalls us by controlling those issues, which are controllable. Remember; place the odds in your favor.

41

Aging

So many folks blow off their ailments, referring to them as just part of getting old. That's certainly the lazy and easy way out. It takes away responsibility for their own health and places it elsewhere. This seems to make them feel better, convincing themselves there is nothing they can do about their predicament. Granted, getting older (as in middle age and above) doesn't usually improve one's health. Instead, it ushers in the process where the machine begins to noticeably break down. It happens to everyone and there's no escaping this bleak reality. However, if your attitude is such that you believe all your afflictions, both the less dramatic variety and those which are potentially terminal, as in heart disease and cancer, are an automatic part of aging, then your opinion that these maladies are inevitable is misguided. Judging by the behavior of the majority of American adults, I would say they subscribe to this defeatist attitude.

Most people believe nothing can be done about their rapidly deteriorating physical condition. Nothing, that is, except for camouflage, diversion and misdirection, which are fake and do nothing to address the infinitely more important underlying problem: their neglectful health behaviors. Humans, by and large, take their health for granted until it's taken away. Then, they worry. A preponderance of individuals are convinced their expeditious spiral to decrepitude is part of the aging process. That it's plainly embodied in the experience. They're satisfied that once they begin getting old, there's no hope. This is not so.

As we enter into the second half of our lives, if we are afforded that privilege, all of our bodies will have begun, years prior, to undergo physiological changes. Changes which irrefutably do nothing to improve our health. Let's face it, we don't see the NFL clamoring to draft too many 80-year-old linebackers. As with any piece of machinery, time and use take a heavy toll. That's why maintenance is a must. You can't stop the deterioration, but it can be drastically diminished.

Think about your body as you would an automobile. Driving it around with the engine constantly at a state of high revolutions per minute and the tachometer always in the red will probably result in a blown engine. The oil must be changed regularly, along with other fluids. Worn brakes and exhaust systems need periodic replacement. Air filters, oil filters, batteries, windshield wiper blades, tires and more all need to be paid attention to and maintained. As the driver of this automobile, you must be mindful of all the systems that it encompasses, in an effort to keep it running as smoothly as possible for as long as possible. Many well-maintained vehicles on our roads have clocked well in excess of 100,000 miles on their odometers. This doesn't happen by accident. When we see one of these vehicles, the reaction is the same as seeing a well-maintained body...wow!

Yes, maintenance is key. Some people will occasionally come across an individual of their vintage who appears years younger by comparison to them. Further, this individual may be in excellent health and makes them look terrible. Many are prone to writing this discrepancy off as nothing more than good luck, good genetics or a good plastic surgeon. Sometimes, they're right. Sometimes, they're wrong. They are few and far between, but there do exist some people who actually care enough about their health to do everything in their power to preserve it, if not improve it. They don't make excuses because they realize that this is the only body they'll ever have to call home. It's a gift and the most important and only place in which they get to live. Setting up their kids for a future of avoidable diseases, as do most Americans, is not what they do. They model appropriate, healthful behaviors for their youngsters and teach them that just because one reaches a more advanced chronological age, which is often beyond our control, does not necessarily indicate that one cannot have a great deal of control as to what that number looks and feels like. Perhaps one day in the distant future, if humanity hasn't yet vaporized itself, we will be swapping out worn, damaged and inferior body parts as easily as we do with automobile parts. That day is not around the corner, only in Hollywood. Until then, it's advisable to keep your own house in order.

Eating well, diligent exercise habits and an overall healthful way of living aren't always the cure-all for every medical problem. Equally, bad food choices and lack of exercise are not the causes of all disease. However, we are well aware that all too frequently, Americans, and in increasingly growing numbers, members of other nations, fall prey to one medical catastrophe or another that would not have befallen them if they'd adhered to a healthful way of life. When it comes to old age, most people, particularly in Western cultures and countries which have adopted a Western culture attitude, never make it to the limits of their genetic potential—physically or mentally.

Great swaths of the rest of the planet are living in abject poverty for a variety of reasons, wondering if they will eat again and be able to find water safe enough to drink. In the majority of the so-called "advanced" nations (technologically speaking, socially remains in question), with their overabundance of food and drink, the bulk of the populace is busily eating for fun, comfort, out of boredom or for a host of other psychologically labeled reasons, rather than putting health and proper nutrition first. Frankly, I find this disgusting. It seems that for nearly every stupid human behavior in today's society, a non-self-incriminatory explanation is unearthed. With these foolish behaviors being encouraged and so eloquently explained away, it's little wonder why so many of us never reach our genetic potential.

Human beings wise enough to engage in the most healthful behaviors possible still become ill upon occasion. The good news is that it's much easier to recover from an illness or an injury as a healthy person, even as a healthy older person. The reason for this is that the body's disease-fighting and healing mechanisms are able to focus on the immediate sickness, as opposed to also having to deal with a half-dozen or so self-manufactured underlying medical afflictions. At best, these will certainly lengthen your recovery time. Further, in an all-to-frequent case scenario, these avoidable, underlying conditions may worsen your immediate illness. Think of it as you would an army with its forces spread too thin because it has been drawn into a multiple-front war. A difficult problem, to say the least.

We are not gods destined to live forever. Regardless of an exceptionally healthful existence, at some point, all human bodies reach their expiration date, including that minority which has attained its genetic potential. The act of living is what ultimately kills us. The mistake is in thinking it's simply the cumulative time spent on Earth that is the enemy. It is not. The true enemy, in the prevailing number of instances, is how we live. What we consider to be "time" is nothing more than a man-made construct. It's a unit of measure we invented to organize and structure our lives. We live in a mostly youth-oriented, fast-moving society. Far too frequently, we give undue credence to this humanly fabricated standard, whereby it is characterized as having a supreme and all-encompassing effect. This belief is unwarranted. We can do nothing about the passage of time as we know it, and obviously, nothing about the concept of what time (for lack of an adequate scientific word) may actually be, if anything. However, we can definitely choose what we do during its passage.

Having lived for many years does not, as a matter of course, define you as old. It simply indicates that you've been around longer than many of your fellow earthlings. If you're in the company of someone who is unfit, with poor posture, needlessly sick and medicated as a result of unwise habits, who complains relentlessly about one nagging malady or another, who is disinterested in the good things which life has to offer, has lost all vigor, who speaks of nothing other than his/her "back in the day" exploits and is generally dour, you're with an old person. Even if that person happens to be only 39 years old.

Conversely, if your companion is fit, stands tall, is free from self-imposed disease, solves problems instead of whining about them, has a variety of interests, is full of zeal, has fond memories but doesn't live in the past because it's more productive to speak of goals and aspirations yet to be attained, is vivacious, content and often quite happy, then, consider yourself fortunate to have someone like this in your life. This individual can most likely teach you a thing or two, although he/she may be 72 years old. This person is young.

The human body is a wondrous, beautiful creation. Most people are blessed with a body free of disease or debilitating health conditions. Unfortunately, early on in life most learn and subsequently adopt the bad habits which our dysfunctional society teaches them. Actions and words demonstrating, encouraging and supporting conduct detrimental to nutritional health and fitness while diminishing or ignoring the ramifications of such conduct abound. They encompass every aspect of our lives, including our homes, schools, places of business, governmental offices, mass media and our social settings. Because deleterious practices are liberally sprinkled throughout the very matrix of everyday life, they go unnoticed or ignored due to their normalcy. These self-destructive behaviors are so ubiquitous that an individual calling them into question is usually described as eccentric. How can a problem that is sickening and killing so many people not register with the population on a grand scale? Because the problem is us, we don't want to hear it, and we're guilty of its normalization. Just as the phrase "all-natural" does not automatically anoint a food product as healthful, so does the word "normal" not make something good, right or just. History is replete with "normal" behaviors.

To greatly improve your chances of aging well, and I'm not simply referring to being able to rise from a chair without the aid of a "crane," you need to dismiss what is normal. Doing so will relegate you to the category of those considered obsessive, compulsive and weird. You will be dismissed as an oddity, but you'll be the one running, jumping, stretching, lifting and laughing as your contemporaries are being wheeled out into the warm, sun-filled dayroom. One needs to have the strength of his convictions and be very strong-willed to face the back of the elevator when everyone else is facing the door.

In this wilderness of the mindless that has become America, where the nutritionally and fitness-challenged reign, well-aged eccentrics are rare, yet they do exist and are marvelous to observe if you come across one. They are having a grand old time and the last laugh while squeezing every drop of juice out of life. This, as they watch the masses, many far younger than they, eating junk, constantly dieting, repeatedly visiting doctors, supporting the pharmaceutical industry, complaining about weight gained over the weekend or holidays, nursing hangovers, and generally following the herd as it is driven like cattle by cultural cowboys.

Partaking of good nutrition and exercise will not empower you with immortality. Good food and exercise may not even add a significant number of years to your life, depending on which research study du jour you choose to believe. What they will do is add life to your years. The more important goal is to increase your health-span. What's the point in living 100+ years if you spend the last half of those years disease-ridden, in pain, immobile and completely dependent upon others? As we age, we become more susceptible to disease and injury as a result of the natural deterioration of numerous bodily systems. Immunity, vision, digestion, the cardio-pulmonary system, the vascular system, the musculoskeletal system and the vestibular system (balance), to name but some of the body's apparatuses, decline in effectiveness the older we get, especially if we advance beyond what is usually considered middle-age, in most cases.

The best-case scenario is to die young but much later in life. Tightly compacting those inevitable years of normally declining health into as few as possible keeps you younger longer. These younger years are your health-span. Of course, the ultimate would be to combine a long lifespan with a long health-span. Short of this, it's probably more advantageous to live less years, the vast majority of them well-lived, and to suddenly die than to live many years, the vast majority of them spent rotting away.

No matter how bad off you are from a medical standpoint, you're more than likely to die sooner rather than later by compounding your illnesses with the ruinous effects caused by unhealthful life habits. It's common knowledge that people who engage in life-promoting behaviors, including excellent nutrition and meaningful exercise and abstain from the destructive practices of eating junk food, drinking alcohol, consuming caffeinated beverages, tobacco use, recreational drug use and roasting themselves in the sun and in tanning beds, dramatically increase the chances that they'll retain their youthful traits longer. They will never look as aged nor suffer from the easily avoidable maladies as their ignorant, uncaring and misinformed contemporaries.

Pot bellies on skinny people, weight gain, dried-out-wrinkled-leathery skin, brittle and prematurely gray hair, blotchy skin, yellow, brittle nails, tooth loss, stooped posture, weakness, fatigue, loss of stamina and overall listlessness, in addition to the potentially deadly diseases I've already mentioned, are not necessarily predetermined harbingers of old age. Sadly, as most of our young people head down the same "fun-filled" road as did their parents before them, we're seeing many of these characteristics in increasingly younger people. Typically, folks begin a physical and mental nosedive as they move past their 20-year high school reunions. Frankly, some don't last that long, the downward spiral having begun at about the 10-year reunion mark. More scientific research isn't required to prove this. Do your own research the next time you're in the local supermarket, mall or any venue where large groups of people gather. Observe the tanning queens who, at 37 years of age, appear to be in their 50s. Take a look at the former star high school athletes who had worked so hard to build up their bodies, only to undo what they'd accomplished. Most of these "glory days" guys in their early 40s look like they're pushing 60. They're done, finished, full of excuses and hopeless. Even the large number of fat grade school kids is staggering. People such as these are the types that encompass the majority of our population. They're fond of saying that you have to live. I couldn't agree more with this sentiment, but the problem is that their idea of living is causing them needless suffering while killing them off early. Adherents to this river boat gambler style of living, more often than not, reap the unnecessary and tragic harvest of the ill-advised seeds they've sown. They've conveniently forgotten that the house always wins. They've squandered or are in the process of squandering their youth while setting themselves up for a very short health span.

On an almost daily basis, one can hear from conversations just how willing so many are to accept their pitiful conditions. They complain about their weight, feeling weak and seem to always be tired. Discussions concerning the numerous medications they ingest are common, again, as if this were a normal part of aging. I suppose that, on some level, it is when you consider that there are more people like this than not. They speak of these pharmaceuticals, explaining how the medicines help them "live with and manage" their numerous conditions. It's as if they're learning to play nicely with someone with whom they don't get along.

I'm convinced most adults are aware that exercise and good food are important constituents of a healthful life. I'm also convinced when it comes to food and exercise most adults are irrational, usually acting in their worst self-interest. You have to search deep within yourself to truly attempt to wrap your head around the idea and fact that one day you will die. Most humans are not wired to deal with their own mortality until it's staring them in the face. By that time, the ravages of heart disease, cancer, diabetes, stroke, hypertension and a myriad of other debilitating and deadly conditions, most often incited by their own delusions, have already done their damage. It's too late.

It doesn't have to be this way. What most Americans view as normal aging is only normal in that it's the prevailing condition. A condition most often resulting from very poor choices. These choices lead the majority not to grow old but instead to spend years corroding and decomposing in place. This is what is supposed to happen when we're dead, not when we're alive. If we decide, the biological realty can be something far better. Chronologically speaking, we can do nothing about the number of years that pass. We can, however, do a great deal about how we pass our years. Being biologically old at the age of 35, for example, and being biologically young at the age of 75 are both attainable. It depends on what our priorities are. Aging is not like jumping off a cliff, where one moment we're young and the next we're plummeting at an ever-accelerating rate of speed into our dotage. Nor is it meant to be a long, torturous, drawn-out process rife with pain and discomfort. We were manufactured to age gradually along a gentle curve. We can live young— running, lifting weights, dancing, hiking and enjoying sex until the end, if we're willing to put in the work. If done the right way, we can remain relatively vital for 99% of our existence and relegate the unpleasantness to the brief remainder.

The well-informed, the dedicated, those who take responsibility, those who realize how precious the gift of health is, the furiously independent who don't give a damn about "what's trending," people not sucked in by slick advertising, those who turn their backs on the fickle, ephemeral dictates of a youth and money-centric culture, these people are the antithesis of those who subscribe to the traditionally accepted version of aging, as determined and defined by society. These are the 70-year-olds who look 56 and act and feel as if they are 45. How can this be? The answers vary. A healthful lifestyle isn't the only answer but it is, without doubt, one of the answers that contributes significantly to aging well.

From the instant a human is delivered kicking and screaming into this world, cosmic forces beyond our inferior human comprehension turn over the hour glass containing the sands of that individual's existence. At this precise moment, the life clock begins to count down, grain by grain, to the inevitable equalizer of all mankind. As I've pointed out repeatedly, nothing can be done to alter our final destination. Despite the belief of some in the scientific community that human life expectancy may someday be infinite, I don't expect that to happen anytime in the foreseeable future. Worrying yourself sick about our ultimate fate will not change it. We can, however, make plenty of prudent decisions along the road which leads us there, increasing our chances of a smoother ride. Unwise decisions, on the other hand, increase the likelihood that the journey will be akin to being violently carsick most of the way.

One's attitude about aging is determined by societal culture, and it is a significant factor in how one lives and, ultimately, how one dies. There are many positive characteristics associated with Western society. Among these are equality, individualism, opportunity and civil rights, etc. The flip side of the Western society coin isn't quite as rosy. Only very strong and committed individuals can turn their backs on the harmful but accepted behaviors of society. Conversely, weak individuals follow these behaviors. They worship youth and money while marginalizing the elderly and the poor. Our society in the west is obsessed with trendiness but never really commits to it because we're always scanning the horizon for the next best thing to come along. We are a capricious lot, gravitating from one inane thing to another for reasons that, at times, defy explanation. In America, what is new, cool, hip and young today is quickly discarded onto the scrap heap of soon-forgotten history. This, as tomorrow's new, cool, hip and youth-oriented interests are hyped by the machines of propaganda. While you're thinking how hip you are for wearing it, driving it, watching it, drinking it, eating it, doing it or being there, the purveyors of these various "its" are laughing at you all the way to the bank.

Have you ever been comfortably seated at home watching an NFL game that was hyped and promoted all week? The game of the season by some accounts. Radio, TV, newspapers and online sources all trip over themselves in order to be the first to report the most innocuous piece of information regarding big, important games. Sometimes, they tell us a game is so big because the speculation is that these two teams will probably meet again in the playoffs. Oh, how the excitement mounts. So, here you sit, Sunday finally having arrived. Your eyeballs are glued to the TV. You don't want to miss one play of this oh-so-important contest. The game commences with the kickoff and the first few plays. You think to yourself that this is going to be a good one. What drama, what excitement—until that is, 4 minutes into this, the supposed biggest game of the year, the announcer reminds you and the rest of the viewers not to forget to tune in next Sunday for that really important showdown between rivals _____ and_____ (you fill in the blanks), a game with

191

important playoff ramifications, and how their network will be broadcasting live from such and such. We are further implored to remember to tune in to the all-important pregame show so that the experts can analyze the analysis with more mind-numbing statistics and blah, blah, blah. Meanwhile, the present most important contest of the season is unfolding before your very eyes as the broadcaster talks over the action, hyping next week's big game.

Wait a minute! Were you not led to believe you are watching the most important game of the year right now? Was not the thrilling prospect of this very game shoved down the collective throats of sports fans all week long? Will you not be permitted to enjoy this game, happening at this very moment, prior to its significance being diminished by the network's hyping of next week's "more," most important of important games? No, you won't be allowed to enjoy the game currently underway because this game is already 4 minutes old—it's just about history! At this point, everyone watching this big game should collectively grab hold of their TVs (get help if it's a theater-sized, wall-hung smart TV) and throw them the hell out of their front windows. I'll keep my TV, switch from the stupid game and watch the History Channel instead. At least I'll learn something.

This "next best thing" attitude manifests itself in a variety of ways. Computers, smartphones, digital and other technological devices, and automobiles are all obsolete by the time you purchase them. So many are swept along with this tide of newer is better. This is in clear evidence as we witness thousands of Americans camping overnight, others rising at zero-dark-thirty to queue up during inclement weather each time a new smartphone is unleashed on the market. They don't have the discipline to wake early for a workout but for the latest phone? Oh yea! No sooner do you acquire the best of the best when the marketing hyperbole regarding the new "best" of the best begins again. So continues the endless cycle of futility.

Let's consider fashion: it's the same pattern of behavior by both the producer and the consumer. Some fashion guru is at this very moment sitting who knows or who cares where, surrounded by sycophants, deciding what trendy, in vogue, must-have articles of clothing and accessories the well-dressed will be wearing six months from now. Never mind that these decided upon fashions will soon go out of—well, fashion. Ridiculously enough, in 20 years or so many of these items will come back into fashion rechristened as "retro." Not too many years ago, kids were wearing bell-bottoms as if this fashion trend was a new discovery. This was exactly what we were thinking in the late 1960s and early 1970s. Little did we realize that sailors were wearing them long before they became a trend and part of the uniform of the counterculture.

Gargantuan houses, sexy automobiles, cool tech, hip clothing, gaudy jewelry, most popular and current catch phrases and words (can we stop saying "awesome" for the so many things that clearly are not?), most in vogue food and drink, most happening hairstyle, must-have accessories and must-see events are all part of the same pathogenic attitude in our society. We are constantly being reminded to "live in the moment" and "be present," along with other lovely, new-age-sounding psychobabble. All this while the majority is running around as if its collective hair is on fire, not wanting to be left out or be caught dead with an outdated item. This seems to me a great way to manufacture needless stress. Our fast-paced culture strikes the match, and we are the fuel. And to what end? One minute, "they" are telling you you belong, and the next minute, "they" announce your irrelevance. How quickly we are deemed yesterday's news.

Our attitudes about aging are but another demonstration of this pathology. Many Americans and many people in general harbor some contorted ideas and viewpoints concerning numerous issues. Screwed-up thinking spawns screwed-up people. This is one reason why so many individuals find themselves broke, uneducated, unfit, with kids who hate them, in jobs they despise and believing the lies and half-truths thrust upon them, on an almost daily basis, by politicians, corporations and the media. We, the people, are inept when it comes to original or independent thought. It's no different when it comes to the topic of aging, whereas most people seem to view it the same way. Doom and gloom.

Most of the people I remember from my high school days have become old, fat farts. They think old, talk old and act old; therefore, they're old. At this juncture in their lives, it seems that there are two predominant topics they can speak about with any positivity and passion. The first is that brief window in their lives, their time in high school when they were hot, buff, cool or athletic. It reminds me of Bruce Springsteen's song, "Glory Days." If they're not boring you to death with tales of their once majestic but now vanished youth, they're lamenting their present state of caducity while elaborating upon the physical decline which transitioning into an older adult initiates in the typical American.

The second of these overriding topics is God. The formerly cool, high school bad-asses have suddenly found God and are reborn as Jesus freaks and Bible thumpers. Don't believe me? Log on to Facebook and take a gander at so many of your former classmates. I can only surmise that the majority are feeling the sands of time slipping away, and they are desperately trying to make amends for their past transgressions. I find it amusing when I encounter high school bullies, dopers, those who disregarded any form of sexual morality because they viewed sex as a competitive sport and those who generally tormented fellow students as well as teachers and administrators, who have the unmitigated audacity to tell the rest of us that the only way to salvation is through Jesus. Amen. The entire tenor of people such as these is gloomy.

High school does not a life make. Stop living your life through the prism of four, forever gone years. What about the rest of your life? What about now? Not to diminish what you may have accomplished in those four years, but if you live in the past, you will most assuredly die there as well. As far as God is concerned, believe or don't, it makes no difference to me. However, as you begin to acknowledge your mortality, don't try to pass yourself off as an enlightened crusader in the army of Jesus. I remember you from high school. These are examples of how you don't want to age.

There exist no laws that state when we reach a certain age, men must wear their trousers pulled all the way up to where their chests used to be or must wear plaid Bermuda shorts with white patent leather shoes and matching belts. Nor is it legislated that men need to allow their nose hair, ear hair and eyebrows to sprout to such an extent that they become wildlife refuges. You're not required to grow man-boobs so they can sit comfortably on your pot belly. Equally, women are not legally compelled to wear stretch polyester pants with old lady shoes. They aren't required to let their sideburns, mustaches and chin whiskers grow to rival those of their mates. The fact that folks have advanced well beyond their high school years into middle age and further is no reason for an ass so fat that it should have its own zip code. There's no reason to be waving at someone and having a large chunk of fat on your upper arm flapping in the breeze. Now, for those of you who actually like these sorts of things, by all means, embrace them. Do them because you want to, not because you've thrown in the towel, or worse because that's what society expects of you.

Older people are not forced to look a certain way, dress a certain way, or get fat, unfit and sick. These are personal choices. If you, as an individual, want to make what you consider to be a change for the better, why give a damn about an overwhelmingly ignorant society's vacillating attitudes? Your attitude about yourself is what matters most. Don't allow yourself to be flung onto the trash heap of soon-forgotten yesteryear. Don't meekly climb onto the miserably pathetic pile of "back in the day." You're still here, you matter. Be the best and greatest you can be right now. Stand up to the trendy and oh-so-hip bullshit produced and advanced by those whose primary interests amount to no more than the emptying of your wallet. Confront those whose slogans, ads and commodities serve little more than to generate and perpetuate the attitudes that make young people old. Do not heed their messages, but listen because knowledge is power, and you must always know the enemy's intent.

Exercise, eat nourishing foods, continue to learn and to challenge yourself. Live, really live, now. Let the worshippers of youth know that by making prudent health choices and with a little bit of luck, they might even have the privilege of reaching your age one day. Getting old is a good thing. It means you're still vertical. Coolness has nothing to do with age. You're either cool, or you're not. Do what you want to do because you want to do it, not because "they" believe you should. The next time some trendy asshole tells you to dress or act your age, challenge him to a run, blow his doors off, and then tell him to go away. Remember, how you age is mostly up to you.

42

Eating And Attitude

Many people who embark on a weight-loss journey are doomed to failure before they begin. This is often due to their single-minded obsession with counting calories. Since they are so focused on the amount of food they consume and its caloric content, they fail to consider what, exactly, they are eating. They spend years talking about their exercise routines and diets and yet complain about the lack of progress. These conversations are especially prevalent during holidays and other celebrations. By way of review, let's revisit Fourth of July barbecues and how they entice the general population to consume popular American standards such as hamburgers, hot dogs, potato salad, chips, beer, soda and ice cream. Afterward, acquaintances commiserate, granting one another absolution for their unwise choices. People are fond of assuaging their own guilt, as well as that of their like-minded associates, by proclaiming they will work-out harder and/or longer to burn off the excessive calories. Yet another method to mitigate guilt for the calorically minded is claiming that they will cut the amount of calories they consume by just eating less of what they've always eaten.

With regard to losing weight, calories do matter, but the belief that simply losing weight is the solution for poor health is without merit. The cultural conversation is all wrong. Yes, being overweight due to overconsumption of calories contributes to a plethora of health problems, but this is only one aspect of a bigger food picture that contributes to poor health in society. Even if you were able to burn off the extra calories consumed during a typical July 4th blowout (you won't) or you were to eat half the amount you usually stuff yourself with at one of these gatherings, the point you're missing is that you're still eating and drinking disease-promoting foods and beverages. While losing weight in the form of body fat may be a box that needs to be checked for most individuals, the attitude that burning off extra calories, eating less food and drinking less is illogical if your diet consists of bad food and drink to begin with. Being a slave to calories and the scale does not necessarily, in and of itself, promote excellent health. Eating and drinking the right types of foods and beverages contribute to excellent health.

When it comes to eating, most American adults behave as children would. Bad food is bad food, not a treat or a reward, no matter the quantity ingested. This fact seems to escape the majority of our population. Kids have a reason for their ignorance; they're kids who need to be taught by

196

logical, rational adults. Sadly, when it comes to eating habits, logical, rational adults are in short supply. Until we stop rewarding ourselves and our children with lousy foods which are culturally labeled as treats, the status quo—that is, avoidable diseases—will reign supreme. Adults who reward children with toxic foods, besides setting their youngsters up for a future of excessive body fat and sickness, are instituting a bad precedent for their children's yet-to-be-born children. In this way, the cycle of nutritional ignorance is perpetuated, becoming ever more entrenched into our cultural norms. We are witness to this today in the U.S. and in many countries around the world. More and more people, adults and children alike, are needlessly suffering from avoidable maladies as a result of tortured logic leading to poor attitudes. Remember that kids learn their behaviors from adults.

If excellent health is your goal as well as the standard you wish to uphold for those you love, then your attitude about the poor foods you eat needs to change. You must see these foods for what they really are, garbage. No sensible person wants to eat garbage, not even a smaller serving of garbage. Until you believe this in your heart and soul, you are destined for a "normal" life, just like the rest of the lost, obese and socially acceptable fat folks, waddling about and wondering why they're sick.

The entire situation is maddeningly stupid. Eating poorly and thinking that you're paying the price for that foolish behavior by walking on the treadmill for an extra 15 minutes is misguided at best. The price you are paying is the damage you're doing to your body by eating poorly in the first place. Working out a little longer or a bit more intensely doesn't make up for polluting the only body you're ever going to have with questionable food choices.

If you eat what is considered by most to be the standard American diet, also referred to as the Western diet, chances are extremely high that you will develop what most consider to be the standard American or Western diseases and ailments. These conditions are also known as the diseases of affluence and are largely preventable. The mostly non-communicable diseases such as heart disease, specific cancers, type II diabetes and the maladies that arise as a result of obesity, conditions which have traditionally afflicted developed nations, are spreading worldwide. One reason may be that as poorer nations develop, the population becomes more affluent and begins to spend money on Western-type foods, which they associate with success. Good marketing promotes this idea.

Most Americans eat a diet low in fiber, rich in fat and high in sugar and salt. When we combine nutritional ignorance, nutritional apathy, processed foods, a penchant for prepared food, fast food, dining out, and any excuse not to cook at home, it's plain to see why the aforementioned eating habits of Americans predominate. It's no joke that the acronym for the standard American diet is SAD.

The majority of the population believes or wants to believe that nothing can be done about standard American diseases, another SAD acronym. They cling to the attitude that these diseases eventually just happen as one ages, that these illnesses are simply an unavoidable part of life. It's this type of thinking that helps perpetuate the woeful state of our health. Our youth pick up on this defeatist attitude, and it greatly influences their decision-making and subsequent actions. It's easy to understand why children pick up where their parents left off. Our food culture is so out of kilter that an alarming number of today's kids are displaying the same "normal" diseases and ailments once predominantly associated with their foolish parents. One would think that if parents truly cared about the health and longevity of their offspring, the alarm bells and whistles would be going off in their heads. The warning would be to not let their kids make the same bad choices that they made. Choices that usually set one up for avoidable diseases, needless suffering, and preventable death. Unfortunately, the only bell going off in the heads of most people is the dinner bell.

Americans interested in their well-being need to change their attitudes about nutrition, fitness and health if they are ever going to stop the avalanche of maladies that threatens to crush them physically, psychologically, and economically. I readily admit that the odds are definitely stacked against the average citizen. This is especially true when one encounters the staggering number of ridiculous manifestations of how society itself aids, abets and encourages its members to go on killing themselves. Countless examples occur on a daily basis in a never-ending assault on our senses from every corner of our culture. It's difficult to make any headway in one's struggle to improve one's health when worthless magazine articles are advising a gullible public that it's okay to eat that extra slice of bacon if you use a little less butter on your fluffy white biscuit. They tell you just what you want to hear.

Mixing and matching substandard foods will help no one attain better health. It's true that if you ate less calories than you burned in a given period, even of inadequate foods like bacon and white biscuits, for example, you'd lose overall weight. There is also a strong probability that you would be fat in terms of body composition. Would you be healthy? No. A quality body runs on quality food. Further, I'll tell you something that those who delude themselves don't want to hear. Don't eat less bacon so that you can eat more butter, and don't eat less butter so that you can eat more bacon. I've got a better idea: don't ever eat either one. Unless, of course, you call into play the "stranded on a desert island" example, and by some miracle, the only edible things are bacon and butter. You're on your own in this situation.

43

Nutrition

Nutrition is the process by which the body ingests food and avails itself of the life-sustaining substances contained within that food. Vitamins, minerals, protein, carbohydrates, fats and fiber are some of these substances. They provide energy for physical and mental performance, serve as a catalyst for cellular growth and support cellular repair. Through nutrition, we fuel our bodies to give us energy to maintain us in top form. The body knows when it requires fuel in the form of food. It makes this need apparent by sending our brains hunger signals.

In a normal person, eating when you are hungry is the way the machine is designed to operate. The human body, requesting nutrients to function properly, needs to be fed to quell the feeling of hunger. When a person eats inferior food for comfort, taste alone, fun, out of boredom, due to anger, as a result of depression, because they are sad (or even happy), habitually or for any of the other muddled reasons people eat, they are not in tune with satisfying the body's natural hunger. In most of these cases, they are doing nothing more than gratifying another desire which has little to do with normal hunger. This is not nutrition, nor does it have anything to do with health and well-being.

Eating is something that most of us engage in each day. For those of us who enjoy being alive, eating as it relates to genuine nutrition is one of the most important subjects we need to master. That most people have such a limited knowledge of proper nutrition is a sad testament to what civilization puts front and center in terms of education. What makes this worse is that countless others take no interest in learning while remaining stubbornly attached to erroneous information and disease-promoting food traditions in a toxic food culture. Tragically, those lost and confused individuals engaged in mindless eating are further encouraged to continue along this deadly path by an enabling society, which endlessly reminds us of the horrific consequences of the obesity epidemic sweeping the land.

It is said that we are what we eat, and it appears to be true. Observe your fellow human beings and see what so many have done to what was once a beautiful work of art and a scientific marvel—their bodies—once filled with so much promise and potential. All those wonderful possibilities and dreams reduced to a disease-ridden, over-medicated, unfit, barely locomotive and prematurely aged reality. The ability and desire to improve our bodies is no less important than the ability and desire to improve our minds and spirits. Actually, all three are interdependent if one is to attain the pinnacle of human development as we know it to be in this time and place. Once you get to the crux of why you're eating, you can begin to improve upon what you're eating.

44

Accountability

It seems to me that as the 2000s began rolling along, so began what is today, a pronounced shift in paradigm seeking to more fully embrace issues concerning cultural sensitivity and rights. Even a casual observer of the world's historical record can clearly discern that humans have an abysmal record of understanding, enclasping and being sensitive to the desires of their fellow humans, whom they view(ed) as different. Any repositioning of the way we think about our fellow human beings, which makes us see them, in fact, as human beings just like us, is a positive step in our evolution. However, it must be noted that as is typical with most changes to accepted cultural norms, the pendulum swings dramatically from one set point to its opposite position before finally settling in a more reasonable place somewhere between the two.

As I write this many state that the sensitivity/rights pendulum needs to remain positioned at its present, historically opposite point, if not further advanced, toward an even more sensitive culture. They argue that this is an effort to balance out the countless instances of repression, discrimination, objectification, domination and overall violations perpetrated upon the more vulnerable members of society by those in positions of power throughout the centuries. Indigenous people, black people, brown people, women, immigrants, the elderly, children, LGBTQ+ people, religious and ethnic minorities, and other groups have routinely borne the brunt of the wanton desires of those in power. These abused groups are angry and have had enough, and I can't blame them.

The opposite take on this subject is held by those who yearn for a return to the "good old days," believing that everything was fine just as it was. People holding firm to this line of thinking, believing that mandated inequality is just, unwilling to see, let alone understand, why their point of view is questionable, are hopeless. We can only hope that these individuals are reduced to an insignificant minority as soon as possible.

A closer examination of these polar opposite ideologies reveals some hybrids. Some groups are of the opinion that change is needed but only champion specific issues. Others welcome radical changes on a combination of sensitivity/equality fronts. Some of these issues include but are not limited to having what they consider to be offensive language contained within classic literature expurgated from their texts, expressing a strong desire to have statues and memorials honoring questionable historical figures removed from the public eye and going so far as to deface or remove the statues themselves, abolishing older cinematic works depicting people, particularly black people, in a negative light and adding gender-neutral pronouns to the cultural lexicon when referring to members of society who identify as non-binary. I get it. I really do, but addressing all these issues would be another book. My purpose for mentioning sensitivity/rights, in short, equality and acceptance, is because the general topic neatly ties into this work's overall theme of well-being. It is to illustrate to you how a good idea with good intentions can become twisted and morph into something harmful. This often happens when we think with our hearts at the expense of our heads.

This discussion about equality and acceptance serves as an interesting segue into the body-positive movement, which has gained significant momentum lately. As a guilty and shame-ridden society attempts to rectify past wrongs, it sometimes overcompensates by creating new wrongs. The furor created by current cultural perceptions of beauty is such an example. The narrative concerning what is considered to be aesthetically pleasing in the human form changes throughout history. From the paintings of fleshy, voluptuous women popularized by Rubens in the seventeenth-century to the thin, androgynous Twiggy-crazed 1960s to steroids-enhanced female bodybuilders of more recent times and every personification in between, perception of the ideal female form changes culturally. The same holds true for males. Fat, wealthy and powerful men of yesteryear were seen as having a presence about them. Enter the likes of Arnold Schwarzenegger and Sylvester Stallone and the popular impression of what constitutes a desirable male physique was turned on its head.

From ancient times to the present, the arts have had a strong and driving influence on what society deems to be an attractive human body. The biggest difference is their level of influence from the past to the present-day world. The advent of modern communication technology has made the sharing of images and ideas voluminous and instantaneous. Information comes and goes much more quickly and reaches a far greater audience. The incessant bombardment of information, much of it bad, upon impressionable minds, provokes their ability to deny reality and create their own reality on a regular basis.

What cannot be denied is that throughout recorded human history, the appearance of real humans' bodies hasn't dramatically changed. What changes constantly is the popular notion of what type of body is in fashion. This has nothing to do with health or reality. Similarly, the tortured reasoning behind today's body-positive, "everyone is beautiful" trend has nothing to do with health or reality. We have choices. We can tell ourselves and our children that the world is beautiful, everyone and everything in it is beautiful, and that everything will be alright. We can deny history by eradicating literature and art. We can censor language and behavior. We can wear cultural blinders while living in a world of make-believe. We can choose to not deal.

The other choice is that we can be honest and deal with reality, something so many people are loath to do. If we were to be truthful with ourselves and our children, we would acknowledge that the world is brimming with a great deal of beauty and wonderful people. However, this is only part of the story. Honesty and reality would compel us to add that if everything were so beautiful, we wouldn't have war, murder, rape, robbery, pedophilia, slavery, genocide, identity theft, fraud, environmental degradation, lying politicians, and so many individuals and corporations inventing new ways to fuck their fellow humans just to make a buck.

Humans are not perfect. I don't believe that every human being that ever perpetrated an atrocity upon his fellow man had a diagnosable condition, a traumatic upbringing or any one of the many excuses utilized to help us understand their horrific acts. Face it, some people are just bad. Furthermore, how alright is everything going to be when death is a certainty in everyone's future? The only alright thing possible is in how you live. After that, who knows?

Absolving those with medical or genetic conditions that cause them to gain weight leaves the vast majority of overweight people who arrived at their present condition through their own behaviors. Within this group are those individuals who are happy in their corpulence—more power to them. Be content in how you choose to live. They should not be shamed or be made to feel less human than anyone else.

My experience has taught me that most overweight people don't fall into the medically, genetically or happily overweight. Most people are overweight because they lack the fortitude to do what it takes to reach a healthful weight. Yes, pornographic food temptation lies around every corner; it feels so good to just lay in bed, exercise is uncomfortable, and our culture is organized in such a way so as to derail our health and fitness efforts. What do we usually do? We give in or make half-hearted efforts that always fail, and then we make excuses, like children. We blame junk food manufacturers, the government, viruses, the media and use whichever excuse happens to be trending.

While it is true that some of these entities are complicit in the deterioration of our health, we permit them too much power. We feebly allow them to control our behaviors, then hold them solely accountable for the consequences of these behaviors. Ultimately, and despite them, we need to take responsibility and be accountable for our own health. We must stop taking the easy way out, including excuses based on lies, bad information, redefining reality, or simply inventing our own reality because it has proven time and again to never work.

We need to be complete in our explanations and meanings. "Everyone is beautiful" makes for a nice, albeit tediously trite meme on social media and is a catchy bumper-sticker. It's also bullshit.

Keep telling your kids this, and they'll be eaten alive in the real world. A 5'2", 300-pound woman in a thong may be educated, have a kind heart and a wonderful personality. No doubt, some might find her physically beautiful. To each his own. She is also, if she hasn't already been diagnosed, at increased risk for hypertension, diabetes, heart disease and a slew of other avoidable and potentially deadly medical conditions. What's so beautiful about that?

In our cultural zeal for inclusivity and sensitivity, exacerbated by a hyper-desire to avoid even the appearance of what might be construed as an offensive deed, word or thought, we've created a dangerously unhealthful environment. People need to be educated about the fact that healthy human bodies, despite their genetically nuanced differences in musculature, bone structure and other such biological characteristics, are generally meant to look a particular way.

The appearance of a healthy human body falls within a wide range of parameters, but there are still parameters. The overweight people we see each day do not fall within these parameters because they've allowed themselves to be accommodated. They've never been taught about the dangerous side of the overweight story in a clear, emphatic, consistent and truthful manner. If society as a whole really cared about each individual, which it certainly does not, education concerning the downside of being overweight would drown out the protestations of the myopic "feel good" crowd.

Ignoring or minimizing the numerous and very real dangers of being overweight and unfit, which I've been pointing out throughout, does a grave disservice to society in general and to our children in particular. The children are in line to be the world's next wave of adults. The world is not in need of another generation of adults with a thumbless grasp of reality.

Most people would agree that education is important. I would concur. However, one of the numerous problems in our education system is that there is a severe paucity of real health and fitness education in our learning institutions. To put it simply, people grow up knowing math, science, reading, writing and the winner's version of history, but they never learn how to properly nourish themselves. They never learn the consequences of a bad diet or how vitally important exercise is at all stages of life. Knowing how to speak well, spell, solve for "x" in an algebraic equation, geography, recall significant historical figures and events, and name all the state capitals is wonderful. These pieces of knowledge are required to more effectively navigate society, including qualifying for and retaining employment.

On the other hand, none of it matters if, due to nutritional and fitness ignorance, you become diseased and drop dead well ahead of your time. I'd rather know how to exercise and eat properly than to have memorized some part of history that we never learn from anyway, are doomed to repeat, and whose telling is tainted by the recorder's agenda. Knowledge of food and fitness keeps an individual alive, but knowing the primary causes of "the war to end all wars," by way of example, will not. Nutrition and exercise education need to be taught with the same, if not a more robust attitude than anything being presented in our schools today. We are in the grip of a completely preventable pandemic of our own stupidity. We don't know what we're doing when it comes to our health or why we're doing what we are doing.

All this ignorance is aided and abetted by a system which talks a good game but ultimately is focused on making money. If we're not being encouraged to "drink responsibly" and eat disease-promoting foods, we're being fed the pablum that being over-fat and out of shape is entirely acceptable and beautiful. I know plenty of fat, unfit people who have beautiful hearts and are generally good folks. This has nothing to do with the fact that they have transformed themselves into unhealthy, grotesque forms of what humans are supposed to be. If they are honestly happy with their condition, good for them. However, let's expand the discussion to include the dangers of carrying around all that "beauty." We are fools being told what we want to hear, being baited and hitting that bait like a school of ravenous fish.

We need to hold ourselves accountable for our own actions. Placing blame elsewhere or torturing reality just to make ourselves feel good is a fool's game. Being over-fat is unhealthy. Being unfit contributes to being unhealthy. That's the simple truth, and it's not beautiful. It's frightening. Learn to deal with it and save yourself and those you love. We need to set the bar just as high, if not higher, for health and fitness through nutrition and exercise, exactly as we do for academics. We need to learn how to eat proper food. We must learn how to exercise so we can increase our chances of a healthful, vibrant life instead of an entirely preventably wretched existence consumed by disease, immobility, doctor's appointments, needless suffering and early death. It's imperative we pass these lessons on to our children.

It is senseless and disingenuous to attempt to rectify a problem only using half measures, partial truths and explaining the problem in such a way that serves a particular group's wishes. The United States of America spends more money on health care than any other country on the planet. Yet, we're one of the unhealthiest and over-medicated nations on Earth. It's no wonder that nearly 75% of our population is overweight. There is a direct correlation between being over-fat and developing some illnesses, particularly those that are preventable. We need to face this fact. We're trying to solve one problem by creating a far worse problem that is endangering our health and lives. We are fat, out of shape, lazy, eat lousy food, guzzle booze, make excuses, blame others for our troubles, lack common sense, lack discipline and will, mismanage our lives and can't handle reality.

To add to this sorry state of affairs, many states are legalizing recreational marijuana so that people's options for escaping reality are expanded. To be clear, I'm not referring to the legalization of medical marijuana to ease the pain and suffering of legitimately sick individuals. No, I'm referring to people utilizing a drug to avoid dealing with the real world. Strong action and a recalibration of what truly matters in life needs to occur if we are to create a whole and healthy society. The truth about what we as a culture are doing to ourselves and setting future generations up for can no longer be relegated to a dark corner. It's time for some plain talk.

45

What To Lose

I've used the term "lose weight" at times because these are the words familiar to most people. However, the goal is not for the "overweight" to simply lose weight but to lose body fat. Burning up lean muscle mass is not the desired outcome. Body composition is more important than body weight. That's where the Body Mass Index (BMI) fails. It is a number calculated from an individual's height and weight which serves as only a fair indicator of the amount of body fat being carried around.

From a health perspective, the calculation doesn't work well on people who are "skinny-fat." Folks in this predicament might actually be lightweights for their respective heights, but they may have a greater percentage of body fat than muscle. The result is that they are skinny in size but made up of too much fat. In cases such as these, it doesn't matter that the scale provides them with an acceptable weight. Unlike their overweight, over-fat friends who cannot hide under a protective layer of garments, these individuals can easily hide their poor physical condition with clothes. Regardless, both groups are unfit.

Through the years, I've known numerous women and men who were too heavy for their respective heights according to the BMI scale. Despite this, they had no weight to lose due to their adherence to consistent exercise and excellent food choices. Their bodies were primarily muscle, which is more dense than fat. One particular friend comes to mind as I write these words. At a height of 5' 7" and weight of 205 pounds, his body fat percentage was less than 10%. This shows us that muscle by volume is heavier than fat.

The BMI scale does not work for these types of people either. You can see why I alluded to BMI not being a very good indicator of what people should weigh. All too often, the bathroom scale is deferred to as the ultimate arbiter when considering one's physical condition. This is a common mistake. The important takeaway here is to understand that it's healthier to be made up of a higher percentage of muscle than of fat. If you're going to lose weight, be sure it's the excess fat weight that you're losing.

People who obsess about losing weight have an unhealthful love/hate relationship with their scales. When the pounds decrease, they love the scale. When the pounds increase, they hate the scale. These people are mainly calorie counters, paying no mind to the type or quality of food they consume. The overall idea of your best health requires much more than simply watching calories and the typically misguided notion of losing weight. You can lose all the weight you want to lose and remain unhealthy and unfit. When it does occur, this kind of mindset renders your weight loss meaningless. If you need to lose weight/body fat, it must be done in an appropriate manner.

For the best health outcome, you need to lose body fat slowly, at a rate of about 2 pounds per week. There are no quick weight loss fixes that are healthful, and that will keep the body fat off permanently. You can be certain of this despite the volume of ridiculous ads to the contrary we see geared towards a desperate and naive public. Weight loss ads are pervasive, especially on social media. They promote quick and permanent weight loss. I recall advertisers claiming that by using their product, customers could lose 30 pounds in 30 days. Even if this claim were true, unless you were morbidly obese and found yourself in an imminent life-or-death situation, it would be most unwise to lose 30 pounds in 30 days. This would be dangerous to your health.

The primary objective is optimal health through permanent lifestyle changes, including proper nutrition and fitness. If this goal is to be realized by those who need to lose body fat, then cutting back on food portions is, in fact, necessary because this will lower caloric intake. Remember, however, that calories alone are only one part of the health equation. The other equally important factor is to permanently and completely remove poor food from your diet. Eat only good food, and exercise religiously in conjunction with your improved eating habits. If you do these things, you'll lose body fat, build lean muscle and ingest significantly fewer toxic substances harmful to your health.

46

Eat At Home

Replacing illness-inducing and illness-exacerbating food with healthful food is not necessarily synonymous with self-deprivation. Look at it as if you are just taking out the trash. It is completely illogical to eat good-tasting food or pseudo-food that promotes disease and also worsens already existing medical issues. What's the point, taste? Is this the singular and all-consuming sense driving your existence? If so, this is, to me, a sign of a very troubled mind. It is children who care only about how good something tastes at the expense of their health, not well-adjusted adults.

Eating yourself into sickness and going through life wearing vertical stripes, dark colors and utilizing other methods of camouflage and distractions to take the focus away from a ruined exterior is no way to live. Once you learn to eat properly by acclimating your taste buds to healthful, nourishing foods, you will no longer feel deprived. Instead, just as you trained your brain to eat harmful foods, you will retrain it to eat health supporting foods and to enjoy them as well. Yes, these new foods will taste good to you. I'm not suggesting that this will be easy, only that the end result will be worth the effort.

If everything in life were fun and easy, we'd all be strutting about with the bodies and faces of Greek gods and goddesses, making and saving piles of money, obtaining advanced college degrees, living for 120 years and being loved by all. This won't be happening. Life is hard, and you usually get out of it what you put into it.

You'll only feel deprivation at the onset of your new way of life. Once you embrace your health and the fat begins to diminish, muscle mass is added, the toxins are excreted, and you become fit, a rewiring of your brain occurs. You will become more enthused as you see and feel the results of a healthful way of life. Many of the foods once viewed as treats and rewards of which you deprived yourself may be remembered as delicious, but these recollections will be tempered with the realization that they are toxic to your well-being and should be avoided. You will learn to love, respect, appreciate and be truly kind to yourself with foods that emphasize your health, as opposed to slowly destroying your life by ingesting detrimental trash, no matter how good that trash may taste.

Taking control of your own life, as much as possible, is one of the keys to an existence of peace and contentment. Taking charge of what you eat is one such aspect of controlling your life. As such, prepare your own meals at home. For the most part, restaurant food, fast or gourmet, is not about health. It's all about taste. Choosing something more healthful from the menu does not mean it's healthful. It simply indicates that it's less harmful than the other item you are considering.

Ordering appetizers only, kid-sized portions or splitting entrées, as some suggest, while certainly diminishing the caloric load of your meal, is only a partial solution. These techniques only enhance the delusion that you're making healthful choices. You, no doubt, will still be consuming needless amounts of sodium, sugar, oils and other unhealthful fats. Obviously, because your portions are smaller, you'll be ingesting less of these, but it's still a roll of the dice where your health is concerned. It's a bad compromise. I don't believe in compromises where my well-being is concerned.

Appetizer-sized meals, kid-sized meals and splitting up portions of less bad food indicate that you are not eliminating substandard food from your diet, only that you are eating smaller amounts of substandard food. Saving part of your meal and taking these substandard food leftovers home does not eliminate the food that is less bad from your diet. Purging bad food and less bad food from your diet is the mission here. Your best health hinges on eating the best food possible.

Most people eat for the wrong reasons, including, but not limited to, eating out of boredom, sadness, happiness, anger, loneliness, self-loathing and so on. This mistake is compounded when not only do they eat for the wrong reasons, but they eat garbage food. Often, even those who eat because they are truly hungry continue to gorge themselves long after their appetites have been satiated. One reason for this is due to the addictive nature, in one form or another, of sugar, salt and harmful fats, which just so happen to be found in abundance in processed, fast, and restaurant foods. Processed foods and fast-food restaurant fare are a significant component of the American diet. Lest you think that dining in a pricey restaurant is indicative of a respite from these harmful ingredients, you'd be sadly mistaken.

Many so-called experts constantly encourage people to enjoy themselves. They suggest to the masses that there is no need for deprivation. These experts suggest that one good solution is for people to eat whatever they wish but to simply eat less of it. As I mentioned a few paragraphs ago, this is not the answer despite what the experts say. This behavior doesn't address the healthfulness of the food, only the amount of calories being consumed. Would these geniuses also advise an alcoholic to just drink a bit less? Would they suggest he consume alcohol in moderation? Would they encourage an addict to shoot just half a syringe of heroin into his vein? How about telling a

211

cocaine user to snort half a line instead of the whole line? Anyone think smoking half a cigarette is healthful? All of my seemingly over-the-top examples sound preposterous, do they not? In fact, they are, but they serve as fitting and cautionary when we're discussing eating foods that induce a precarious health outcome. If you care, I mean really care about your health, you don't ever endanger it by eating bad food, not a little bit of it, not in moderation. You don't eat it—ever.

Eating a nourishing and balanced diet means eating a variety of the best foods available. It does not mean balancing the best foods with the worst foods. This is plainly stupid. Learning to prepare your own meals at home by using the most healthful ingredients can be a life saver. This allows you to choose exactly what you want to eat and to control what you do or don't add to your food. Take an interest in learning how to cook. It's not difficult. All that's required is some rudimentary knowledge. You needn't be a chef or have obtained a PhD in nutrition. If I was able to learn, anyone can. Do a little research and teach yourself about the roles that basic nutrients play in fueling the marvelous machine that is your body. Be patient with yourself insofar as you must realize that you have been indoctrinated into and have existed in a culture of systemic malnutrition for your entire life. Learning how to recognize, choose, prepare and enjoy delicious, healthful food is a new chapter in your life. You don't have to make an overnight transformation. It may take a bit of time, but the important thing is to begin building a new healthful foundation that will ultimately carry you through the rest of your life.

47

Diet And Prehistoric Man

The word "diet" was originally defined as the food and drink routinely consumed by human beings and other living organisms. Later, it took on other meanings, including "restricted eating in order to lose weight." When the word diet is used today, more often than not, people immediately think of the latter definition: losing weight by means of calorie restriction. Presently, it seems that nearly every American is on one sort of trendy diet or another. The result of all this dieting is that we have become fatter than ever.

Prehistoric man didn't need to diet, nor did he stress about not being able to find time to exercise. He was too busy merely trying to get through the day in one piece. More likely, he was too busy trying to survive the next hour. Who needs the gym when you're spending nearly all your waking hours running after food and then engaging in a life-or-death battle with that potential food in order to subdue it? As if all that physical activity were not exhausting enough, primitive man's remaining time was devoted to the avoidance of becoming the main course for some ferocious diner. All this expended energy kept him in pretty good shape. However, his good shape wasn't about looks; it was about function. Being able to function in order to simply survive was the goal.

Prehistoric man undoubtedly consumed a far more healthful diet than modern man. Everything was organic. Earth was not yet tainted by the overwhelming amount of environmental pollutants with which we've senselessly poisoned her. There were no chemically processed fake foods. Our ancestors ate plants, fruits, nuts, seeds, roots and game; it was a diet high in fiber, carbohydrates, fat and protein. They got plenty of exercise and had a healthful way of eating. This was a simple formula for success.

What happened? Why is modern man so fat? One reason is due to the incompatibility between natural survival and being thin. We've all known overweight people who have dieted to lose weight. Usually, they initially lose weight by eating smaller portions or by missing meals, thus restricting calories. Years ago, I had an over-fat coworker who wouldn't eat all day. After work, he would go home and eat a big dinner. At first, he lost weight. Soon after, he plateaued and ended his calorie-restricting diet. Not long after this, he began to gain back the lost weight, regaining it all. In addition to this, he gained more weight. As if this was not enough of a problem, it was also plain to see that his body composition had deteriorated. He would frequently complain that he couldn't understand how he was getting fatter with all the dieting he was doing.

His foolish way of eating had forced his body into survival mode, a vestige of our primitive lineage. During the times of prehistoric man, it was either feast or famine. Every so often, his food supply, due to circumstances beyond his control and the indifferent proclivities of nature, would become severely diminished to the point of threatening his very existence. When food, hence calories, became scarce, ancient man's body would automatically go into survival mode. This was essential in order for him to live, but is problematic for modern man.

Based on individual physiology, each human requires a certain number of calories in the form of food on a daily basis to maintain body mass. Over time, weight loss occurs when this caloric intake drops below what the individual's needs are. This holds true during real or self-imposed conditions of calorie restriction. The weight, or body mass that is shed, is in the form of fat and muscle. The body will usually discard more muscle than fat because it knows that more calories are required to preserve muscle than to preserve fat. This is the body going into survival mode. Because this survival mechanism is triggered due to the body recognizing that less calories are being ingested, it initiates the process of storing more fat for survival during future episodes of food scarcity.

Sooner or later, food becomes available again, and all is well. However, the body has now been programmed to remember that sometimes food is in short supply. It needs to make preparations and take precautions in the event that famine strikes again. This is done by storing fat, which is easy to put on and maintain. On the other hand, vanquishing unneeded, dangerous fat requires quite a struggle for modern man.

Today, we impose artificial famines on ourselves through diets just to squeeze into swimsuits. Once we perceive ourselves to be swimsuit-ready, having lost the predetermined amount of weight, we resume our normal, unhealthful manner of eating. Our bodies and nature don't know or care if we are cavemen or modern men. A natural organism instinctively wants to survive. As far as it's concerned, it senses famine and ultimate starvation. The body remembers each episode of on-and-off dieting. Each time we diet, commonly known as "yo-yo dieting," the body loses more and more muscle in addition to fat. At the end of our diet, the body has accumulated even more fat. At this point, we are actually in worse condition aesthetically, as well as from a health standpoint, than when we started all the dieting.

A life of on-and-off dieting is harmful to numerous body systems, including the slowing down of metabolism. Muscle burns more calories than fat. By losing more and more muscle through dieting, the body adds more and more fat. The result is your body naturally burns less calories than before. Besides transforming yourself into a misshapen, blubbery mass as a consequence of your dieting, you need to realize your old fat and your newly accumulated fat are doing a lot more than just clinging to you and making you look—well, fat.

All your fat is as alive as the rest of you. It requires nutrition. As such, if you are carrying around more than the necessary amount of body fat for healthful body operation, this excess fat lures nutrients away from other parts of your body that legitimately need them. This extra adipose tissue expels toxins into your body as a result of its own metabolism. It negatively impacts your hormones and squeezes internal organs, thus debilitating their ability to properly function.

Extra body fat is harmful enough, but worse if it's situated around your belly. It's common knowledge that those with higher concentrations of belly fat increase their vulnerability for cardiovascular disease, diabetes and certain cancers. Although, I recall reading that some have suggested it doesn't matter if you're a fat "apple" shape or a fat "pear" shape—both body-fat types are equally injurious to your health.

For most people, the proper, wise method to lose excess body fat while maintaining a healthful body weight is to eat 3 or 4 healthful meals each day. This roughly and loosely translates to eating about every 4 hours or so. Dieting and becoming famished will only cause you to gorge yourself when you finally do eat. Despite the fact that you have not eaten all day, much of this gorged food will be stored as fat by your survival-mode body. The moral of the story is that if your goal is to get fatter, go on a diet. You've got to eat properly to shed unwanted pounds.

48

Trendy Diets And Practices

Zone, South Beach, Sonoma, Best Life, Atkins, Ornish, Cabbage Soup, Raw Food, Three-Hour, Blood Type, Personality Type, Calorie Restriction, Pritikin, Mediterranean, High Protein, Pescatarian, Macrobiotic, Grapefruit, 80-20 (or Weekend), No Carbs and on and on ad nauseam goes the list of "sure-fire" diets. These are just a smattering of the never-ending, and constantly being added to, list of diets that we as a nation attempt in our ceaseless, failing battle of the bulge. We are a pitiful country of suckers as we jump on the latest diet fad. Add to this trendy list the celebrity secrets to losing weight touted in supermarket rags, plus our own screwy methods such as fasting, drugging, smoking, use of laxatives, cleanses, generally starving ourselves and obsessively exercising to the point of diminishing returns, and it's clear that diets aren't getting the job done. The result of all our dieting is a mostly fat, miserable population desperately searching for the next weight-loss miracle. We refuse to accept the fact that 3,500 calories have to be burned to lose 1 pound of body weight. We are loath to change our stupid eating habits, the very ones that make us sick.

People don't want to hear about desire, commitment, work or will. They literally want their cake and are certainly eating plenty of it. Where weight loss is concerned, the masses want to hear about something easy, catchy, new or fun. That's one of the reasons we see an uptick in promises to drop weight every year on New Year's Day. It's fun to jump on the bandwagon and make meaningless resolutions. We try what celebrities say they do to stay thin. We believe them when they tell us they never work-out, eat what they want or that they're genetically blessed. If any of these Hollywood types told us the truth about how they became fit—consistent exercise and eating properly (the ones who actually do)—most people would tune them right out. The celebrity and diet magazine industries would disappear.

Celebs are like the rest of us. They are only people. Some make good health choices, while others choose poorly, just like the rest of the population. People want magic and instant gratification. In this way and many others, they are childlike. I'm sorry, but reality being what it is, becoming healthy and fit through exercise and body-fat loss don't qualify for instant gratification, and there is definitely no magic involved. You didn't become a whale overnight, and you sure as hell aren't going to be a minnow by tomorrow. You need patience, determination and commitment. It's that simple. I know this isn't what you want to hear, but that's the truth, and it's about time you accepted it if you are serious about a healthy you. You must change your lifestyle, making your health your priority. Anyone telling you anything else has another priority that does not involve you.

Dieting is a mistake. It's foolish and a waste of time and effort. Dieting can be compared to what happens to the vast majority of people when they clean out a closet. It stays clean for a while, but inevitably, due to a lack of discipline, people return to their old habits. They start accumulating and shoving junk back into the closet again. They remain in an endless, fruitless cycle of cleaning and accumulating, like up and down dieting. They refuse to learn from their repeated mistakes.

Thinking about losing excess body fat and being honest about your desire to do what it takes go hand in hand. Are you ready to adopt a new way of looking at things that will lead to a change in the way you live? If the answer is no, then you will be doomed to failure, as in the above-described closet example. Eating a certain way may result in initial weight loss, but remember, your best health is not determined solely by weight loss through calorie counting. While expending more calories than you ingest is the simple explanation for weight loss, eating certain foods and not eating others is the key to optimal health, which is easily within your grasp if you so desire. This is the most significant aspect of healthful nutrition with which the majority can't seem to come to terms. You can be skinny and unhealthy, too.

Ignore the weight loss fads and trends. Stay away from the pills, potions and wacky gadgets. A simple online query will unearth numerous unscrupulous merchants who aggressively market weight loss pills that don't do what their promoters state. Deceptive advertising happens all the time because the manufacturers of these useless products know that there are just enough desperate, gullible and delusional people around to keep their profits rolling in. These liars depend and count on your weaknesses.

Why would you believe a celebrity who says he or she attained that body by taking a particular pill? Do you believe it's gospel because it's stated by a celebrity? Many companies pushing diet-magic use Photoshop and other methods of visual subterfuge to improve the appearance of their models. In addition to retouching photos, many of the physical improvements shown in advertisers' "before and after" pictures credited to their secret pills are nothing more than tricky models doing their jobs. It's obvious that so many of them had a good physical foundation to begin with, but some gained weight for the "before" shots of themselves.

These people know how to begin dropping unwanted weight when the photography sessions end and, no doubt, quickly return to their regular workouts and proper nutritional habits. Many also use poor posture while posing, emphasizing rounded shoulders and protruding bellies, giving the illusion that they are in worse condition than they really are.

Drugs—even if FDA-approved for weight loss, diets, gadgets and gimmicks are a fool's road on the journey toward the healthful and successful shedding of body fat. However, it's important that I repeatedly stress I am not referring to individuals under a doctor's care, morbidly obese people, those who have serious health complications or whose lives are in danger due to one medical condition or another. I'm addressing myself to the majority of the overweight and unfit population, of which the aforementioned group is but a fraction. I would generally advise these people to stick to what works best, exercise and eating right. Don't get seduced into weird idiosyncratic behaviors that people fall prey to, believing they are the secret that no one ever told them about losing weight and acquiring excellent health.

For example, a guy at the gym told me he never eats fruit because of its high sugar content. This is a mistake because the upsides of eating fruit—vitamins, minerals, fiber and other nutrients—far outweigh the negative effects of the naturally occurring sugar in fruit. Eating fruit is a far cry from consuming commercially produced candy bars, cakes, snacks and soda.

49

Idiosyncrasies

As noted before, many people display an inability to deal with reality. As a result, they seek out seemingly fast and easy fixes for their weight and fitness problems. These fixes always end the same way, in failure and frustration. Advertisers depend on our vulnerability. They use keywords in their pitches to elicit public behaviors which will ensure them a profit. Most people like to hear words such as quick, easy, convenient, natural, cheap and so on. Our mostly lazy nature usually overrides our common sense and any innate feelings we may have that we're being fleeced. We so want to believe that becoming healthy and fit is exactly as it is presented to us by those pushing their products and techniques. They readily oblige by telling us exactly what we want to hear. It's tantamount to telling a child that Santa Claus, The Easter Bunny and The Tooth Fairy are real. We all want to believe.

Of course, there are also those practices that some people come up with, from whence I do not know, that are purportedly "health secrets." Many of these nuggets of useless information routinely make the rounds in gyms and health clubs, where they are enthusiastically shared by the believers. As a result, they graduate from being secrets to becoming gospel. This is most unfortunate. If the receivers of these canons of well-being actually took a good look at the physical condition of the vast majority of the dispensers of all this sage information, they would seek more credible sources.

I've been told by some gym gurus that one should never eat past a certain hour of the day. Six-o'clock seems to be the most popular time to stop eating for those adherents of this particular mandate. They believe eating after this hour will cause them to become fat. Yes, going to bed on a full stomach can be quite uncomfortable and may inhibit proper sleep. However, the reality is that it's not the time of day you eat that's the problem. It's how much and what you eat that makes you fat. Calories don't care what time it is.

Some people believe frozen vegetables to be far inferior to fresh vegetables. If you pick them from your garden and eat them soon after, they probably contain more nutrients than in any other form. The vitamin and mineral content begins to degrade the longer they are stored. Frozen vegetables, on the other hand, keep most of their nutritional value because shortly after harvesting, they are quickly frozen, securing their nutrients.

Many individuals have jumped on the "organic only" bandwagon. Many people who claim to eat only organic foods are very fat. I see them at grocery stores like Whole Foods with alarming regularity. However, eating organic is only one aspect of an overall healthful way of life. These folks are obviously neglecting the other, more significant aspects of a well-rounded health regimen. Organic food is not significantly more nutritious than food grown utilizing standard methods. Organic, in its purest form, means the food was grown without certain chemicals being applied, which is a health-positive thing. From a health perspective, organic is unquestionably the better choice. There is nothing healthful about ingesting pesticides, herbicides or fungicides. I'm not interested in the assurances of some governmental authority regarding the GRAS (Generally Recognized As Safe) amounts of poisons being applied to my food. If you can't buy organic because your store doesn't carry it or you've been priced out of the market (organic is more expensive), don't despair. As I mentioned above, organic is but one aspect of a healthful way of life. Make sure you thoroughly scrub and rinse your non-organic produce in cool water. As a reminder, organic junk food is still junk food.

Certain individuals claim physical activity is a mistake and a waste of time for those seeking to shed unwanted pounds. They believe not exercising will help a person lose weight because exercise makes people hungry. The theory goes that if you exercise, you'll consume even more food than you did when you didn't exercise. The more calories you burn up, the more calories you'll ingest later, or so they profess. Advocates of this method of weight loss believe that the only dietary change needed is taking in less calories, nothing more.

At this juncture, some nuances come into play. Generally, it's true that consuming less calories than you expend will cause you to lose weight. Remember, however, the excess weight we want to lose is body fat, not muscle mass. Again, this attempt at wellness is narrowly focused on only one sliver of overall health: losing weight. This focus on simply losing weight is shortsighted, failing to embrace what should be an all-encompassing goal of total health improvement.

Regimented and consistent exercise reduces the risk factors associated with heart disease, vascular disease, certain cancers and diabetes. Exercise may make you hungry, but it's how much and what you eat that is important. Many of the overweight people I've observed in gyms can't wait to reward themselves with bacon, eggs, home fries, buttered white toast and a couple of cups of coffee at the local diner after their morning workouts. That's why they're overweight, not because they exercise. The problem lies in their food choices.

People subscribe to hundreds if not thousands of beliefs, theories and practices when it comes to health, nutrition and fitness. There are those who swear that taking vitamins allows them to eat whatever they want. Some claim to eat "all-natural" while failing to realize the existence of an entire universe of "all-natural" junk food. Some folks exercise for the sole purpose of denying themselves nothing that they can fit into their mouths. I've spoken to yoga practitioners who contend that yoga covers it all as far as health is concerned. Yoga is wonderful, but if your diet is lousy, you do no cardio or strength training, it's far from enough. Cardio without strength training is incomplete. Strength training without cardio is equally lacking.

I've spoken with people whose diets were typically poor and exercised haphazardly, if at all. Nevertheless, they brimmed with confidence that their periodic ritual of colon cleansing was the key to a healthy body. Some of these individuals were of the "do it yourself" school, whereby they would purchase supplements such as laxatives in the form of powders, pills or specific herbal teas and take them orally. These types of supplements induce the colon to empty its contents.

I was surprised to discover that among those individual adherents of colon cleansing with whom I spoke, the majority were not "self-cleaning" but visited a person who cleans colons for a living. The practitioner irrigates your colon with about 20 gallons of water through a tube inserted into your rectum. The fluids and waste are then flushed out through another tube. Water pressure and temperature are sometimes varied. Sometimes, practitioners add nutritional supplements to the water flush.

People undergo these procedures in the belief that undigested food builds up in the colon, producing toxins that pollute the blood and, hence the body. They further subscribe to the theory that these toxins cause a variety of conditions, including, but not limited to, weight gain and fatigue. Individuals who practice colon cleansing advise that it rids the colon of significant amounts of putrefied, presumably poisonous effluent, which routinely sticks to the walls of the colon. By doing this, they feel they can control their weight, reduce the risk of colon cancer and bolster their immune systems.

Those who disagree with this practice believe that normal bowel movements are sufficiently effective in cleaning out the colon. The body doesn't require this extra procedure because normally occurring good bacteria living in the colon detoxify waste, as does the liver. The colon is lined with mucous membranes that keep harmful materials from being absorbed by the body. In addition, the colon discards its old cells every few days, thus precluding an accumulation of harmful matter.

Colon cleansing, as with everything else in life, involves some risks. I'm no doctor, but the difference to me is that some risks are necessary and worth it, while others are questionable at best and unnecessarily dangerous at worst. No government agency oversees colon cleanse products, so you have no safety guarantees. Each state has its own licensing requirements for colon cleanse businesses. Potential risks include nausea, cramps, dehydration, vomiting, bowel perforation, infection and possible allergic reaction if the practitioner adds supplements to the irrigation water. Frequent practice of colon cleansing can ruin the balance of healthy bacteria in the colon. It can also impair normal bowel function.

Call me crazy, but in my estimation, a diet rich in fruits, vegetables, whole grains, beans, nuts and seeds, all of which are good sources of fiber, is a far more reasonable way to improve not only the health of your colon but of your entire body. Along with drinking plenty of water and proper exercise, this type of diet is one of the facets to achieving overall excellent health. You can flush out your colon as much as you like. If you do not eat properly and exercise, it won't make a difference.

Another interesting behavior whose more zealous adherents claim is a panacea for all that ails you is oil pulling. This is the practice of mouth swishing and pulling through the teeth an edible oil, such as olive oil or coconut oil, for a prescribed number of minutes and then spitting it out. It is claimed that this behavior is good for oral hygiene due to the bacteria-killing properties of the oil. Coconut oil is especially popular among oil pullers. Oil pulling is viewed as part of alternative medicine and originates from Ayurvedic medicine. It is said to be good for all matters pertaining to oral health, including eliminating bad breath, healing diseased gums, preventing tooth decay and whitening teeth.

There isn't enough research on the subject to substantiate these claims, but some people are believers nonetheless. I've never tried it. I keep it simple by brushing, flossing and getting regular dental examinations. Of course, if you do some simple online checking, you'll find all sorts of folks claiming that oil pulling is not only good for oral hygiene but that it can detoxify the body, cure diabetes, reduce allergies, help fight cancer, improve acne and a host of other wonderful things. Maybe, maybe not. As I stated, there is no scientific evidence to support these varied claims.

I've spoken with some people who practice oil pulling, who were not regular exercisers, consumed alcohol and coffee, and whose diets were poor. When I tried to question them about their other less-than-stellar health habits, they nimbly avoided these questions and steered the conversation back to the all-encompassing benefits of oil pulling. To them, that is the essence and the secret of good health.

People who engage in these particular and supposedly health-minded practices, each claiming that his specific behavior is the ultimate one for ensuring good health, have one thing in common—they all avoid the gigantic pink elephant in the room that represents good nutrition and exercise. Some of these very specific habits are, in fact, beneficial when examined on their own. Eating organic foods is of obvious benefit. Other habits, such as not wanting to eat after 6:00 pm, are benign. Some habits can adversely affect your health, the complete opposite of what you're trying to accomplish. Finally, certain behaviors have me shaking my head in despair at the utter gullibility and rampant stupidity displayed by the masses who take health advice from supermarket rag sheets and questionable social media sites.

People who are as healthy and fit as they can possibly be do not subscribe to just one of the narrowly scoped behaviors outlined above. They understand that the key is to put as many worthwhile behaviors together into one sensible package. Overall, very few have yet to grasp this concept or at least put it into practice. Simple is usually best. Instead of wasting precious time scouring the internet for obscure and miraculous solutions to your health and wellness problems, the answer is as easy as committing to an exercise program—now. Walk briskly (a relative term) for 3 minutes away from your house, then turn around and walk back home. You just did cardio. It's a beginning. Too much for you? Do 1 minute if that's all you can handle. The point is you don't need anything or anyone to do this, just your desire. Do it every day. In conjunction with this exercise program, commit to NEVER drinking soda again (unless you're near death from dehydration during an apocalyptic event and there's no water available).

It is often said that the longest and most arduous journey begins with the first step. However, this first step must be made while you're pointed in the right direction. It is easy to get pointed in the wrong direction and suffer the consequences of wandering around aimlessly, forever, never reaching your goal. The first step toward excellent health and fitness is to realize that exercise and nutrition are, together, an inseparable marriage. Then, put this realization into practice as described in the previous paragraph's example. Always start with eating and exercise (cardio and body-weight training) to improve your physical well-being. The nuanced knowledge will follow. Then, the more positive behaviors you can weave into your life, the better results you'll get for your efforts.

As you begin to grow into a fit and healthful way of life, you must make sure to avoid the temptation of resting on your laurels. Always seek improvement. Science changes. New discoveries are made. Listen and learn about what's going on in the world of nutrition and exercise. I don't mean that you should jump on every whacky bandwagon out there, and we know there are plenty of those. Learn to filter the information.

If you hear words such as miracle, easy, no sweat, secret technique and the like, it's usually quackery. Further, keep it simple. Throughout the many years I visited gyms scattered about the United States, I usually encountered a handful of individuals attempting intricate, convoluted, unnecessary and often dangerous exercises. More specifically, exercise modifications. I doubt if their reasons for modifying these exercises were because the original iteration of the exercises were too easy for them.

More than likely, they felt that performing these movements made them look very learned and superior to the rest of the gym members. A favorite example is those individuals climbing backwards on stair-climbing machines. Stair-climbing machines, when done in the traditional front-facing way, standing upright, and not draped over the top of the machine, are challenging enough for the most fit individuals. It's relatively easy to slip off the steps and sustain an injury while doing the exercise as it was initially intended. Performing the exercise facing backwards, unless you're training for a circus act, adds needless risk. There is no need to reinvent the wheel in this case. Use common sense, think critically. Put in the exercise work and begin improving your diet. Most of the rest is just noise.

While you're improving your diet and expanding your exercise program, don't forget to begin eliminating unhealthful behaviors and foods from your life. Embrace as many healthful behaviors as possible. After a while, this manner of thinking becomes automatic. Do so at a pace that is within your comfort zone, but don't wait for "someday." We only have so many heartbeats. No matter what you may hear, the foundation for improving your health and fitness is sensible nutrition, cardio, strength training, stretching and balance exercises. If you wish, for example, to take yoga classes or study tai chi in an effort to build upon this foundation, I strongly encourage you to do so. If you play tennis, basketball, enjoy gardening, great. Partake in all these activities after your workout, not in lieu of it. If you insist on having your colon irrigated after this, you're on your own.

50

Some Americans

Some Americans are aware they carry an unhealthful amount of body fat. Some Americans carrying an unhealthful amount of body fat are delusional, believing they are fine just as they are. Some Americans carrying unhealthful body fat claim to want to improve their health. Some Americans carrying unhealthful body fat couldn't care less about their health because their prime directive is to eat now and think about what they will eat shortly thereafter. Some Americans carrying unhealthful body fat regularly exercise and diet, while making sure to reward themselves with treats and cheat meals because of their diligent efforts.

These particular individuals are befuddled as to why they can't "exorcise" their unhealthful body fat. Some Americans carrying unhealthful body fat are vegetarians and vegans, eating only organic and all-natural products. Some Americans carrying unhealthful body fat swear by holistic methods to improve and maintain wellness, eschewing all other modalities. Some Americans carrying unhealthful body fat consume weight-loss pills and other heavily promoted magic potions in a vain attempt to shed unwanted pounds. Some Americans carrying unhealthful body fat purchase fancy abdominal exercise devices, as seen on TV. All these people will continue their life's journey along with their ever-present companion, unhealthful body fat.

Some thin Americans are under the sadly mistaken impression that because they are thin, they are healthy and fit. They don't give health and fitness a second thought. Some thin Americans want to improve their health, generally. These are the ones who realize that thinness does not necessarily equate to being healthy. Some thin Americans couldn't care less about their health because they're thin, life is a party, and they subscribe to the old adage, "If it feels good, do it." Some thin Americans, like their brethren carrying unhealthful body fat, call themselves vegans or vegetarians and eat organic and all-natural products. These are among the thin Americans interested in health improvement. Even so, many of these supposedly health-aware thin Americans have poor diets. Some thin Americans want to bulk up (young male athletes usually come to mind), but when they do, they become fat Americans.

As I pointed out earlier, some thin Americans are also fat Americans. While they aren't bursting out of their shorts, their body composition is too high in fat in relation to their body's lean muscle mass, bone and water makeup. This is why, all too often, body weight alone is a false indicator of an individual's health. By way of review, what your body is made of matters most of all. There are many people hiding beneath their clothing, putting forth the illusion that they are fit when the reality is they are far from it. All of these people remain skinny-fat Americans.

Basically, despite at least a rudimentary knowledge of nutrition and fitness, the majority of Americans, those carrying unhealthful body fat, as well as the thin, educated or uneducated, are one large mass of misinformation and confusion. This misinformation—and even good information—becomes more convoluted with each passing day. Confusion and mistakenly held beliefs concerning nutrition and fitness do not discriminate on the basis of race, gender, ethnicity, religion, age, sexual orientation, wealth, political affiliation or any other socio-economic group you can think of. You need only take a good hard look around. Rich, poor, black, brown, white, Asian, women, men, children, LGBTQ+, intellectuals and idiots—Americans all—have one thing in common, they are in poor physical condition. This includes those who adhere to what they believe is some sort of health practice.

51

Fat Pets And Their Humans

Excess body fat is dangerous to one's health. This isn't just my opinion but a scientifically and medically proven fact which has become common knowledge. I recognize this may not be newsworthy to some. Yet, with foodies pushing their epicurean agenda, sensitivity and political correctness sometimes running amok, it necessitates I point out the obvious. I'm not body-shaming, so let me launch this preemptive strike right now. Over-fat is the predominating health problem in this country and, increasingly, the world. It's a convenient cop-out by those who can't deal with reality to label someone pointing out a health problem as a body-shamer. This type of labeling diminishes a life-and-death issue by diverting the conversation and cloaking it in a mantle of sensitivity-speak. Behavior such as this actually impedes progress toward people becoming healthy. They are more apt to listen to a tender story about their feelings than to the naked truth about them killing themselves through their own stupidity. Body-shaming helps no one. On the other hand, a good dose of reality forces people to see things they would otherwise avoid. This attitude won't make me the most popular guy at the party, but I'm not here to win a popularity contest.

America's over-fat problem has become like one of those horrendously deadly wildfires that happens every year in western states. It's out of control, often kills people and is nowhere near being contained. The main reason this country is so fat is because adults pass on the same behaviors that caused them to become fat to their children. Adults don't take care of themselves, nor do they take care of their offspring. As if this isn't bad enough, it appears they don't take care of their pets either, primarily their dogs and cats. Adults make themselves, their kids and yes, even their pets fat. Unless you have an unusually intelligent pet who reads, comprehends what he sees on TV, understands advertiser's pitches on the radio, and is otherwise social media savvy, plump cats and dogs are victims, but not of big corporations. They can point their furry paws directly at their humans for allowing them to get fat. Hell, we even over-feed our goldfish. Americans have thrown in the towel on themselves, their kids and their hapless pets.

People refer to their animal companions as family members. It then stands to reason that their behaviors mirror those of their owners who are the responsible members of the household and charged with their care. The same questions we should be asking about ourselves should now be asked about our porcine pets. Should we feed them less food? Should we feed them more healthful food? Do they need exercise? Do they require snacks? Well, not necessarily. We can offer the same solution to our chubby pets that we offer to dietarily out-of-control humans—magic elixirs. If one performs a simple online search, one will discover a profusion of dog and cat diet pills. I'm not kidding. This would actually be hysterically funny if it wasn't such a sad testament to what we've become as a society.

Since most of human society has given up on eating and exercising properly, pets don't stand much of a chance. If the concept of eating healthfully and working out happens to register on people's mental radar, it's no more than an insignificant blip on a screen cluttered with lousy food choices and vapid social media memes.

Humans, like water, usually seek the path of least resistance. The pervasive idea that pills and powders are the easy way to lose unwanted weight remains entrenched in the public's mind. It's more palatable for many to think this way than to consider the work required for meaningful lifelong change. This leaves the desperately overweight at the mercy of far too many unscrupulous weight-loss supplement makers, whose claims of miraculous body transformations are without merit. The FDA (Food and Drug Administration) has its hands full chasing these heartless swindlers around. The desperately overweight are reduced to nothing more than victims waiting to happen.

For some individuals, bariatric surgery is the answer. This is major surgery and a chancy operation at that. Even pre-teens are getting their stomachs banded or stapled. Unfortunately, many individuals who have gone through this procedure failed to follow their physician's advice regarding exercise and diet. Whether you want to accept it or not, it always comes back to exercise and diet. As a result, many regain weight, some actually surpassing the initial weight that drove them to bariatric surgery. I've personally encountered a number of people who fall into this category. I suppose there are some people so far gone who require this type of operation as a last-ditch effort to save their lives. Too bad for them that we don't live in a world where health is cherished, even when you have it. With all the dangerous, foolish and debilitating behaviors that we, as human beings, become indoctrinated into, a beneficial indoctrination would be one that began at birth, instructing us on how to eat, exercise and lead a life of overall health and fitness. This would truly serve our species, as well as the environment and all other living things. It would provide a much better solution for weight loss if we didn't need such a dramatic solution for weight loss.

You've seen the pictures. Many of the larger bariatric surgery patients, depending on their personal health histories, habits and other factors, are left with copious amounts of excess skin once they reach a more normal weight. Many opt to have this excess skin removed through plastic surgery, increasing their odds of infection and other surgery-related complications. Others choose to avoid further surgical procedures and instead hide their folds of hanging skin by wearing compression garments. It strikes me as exceedingly sad that a person has to initially deal with a deadly situation and is then forced to deal with a self-esteem issue caused by rectifying his or her life-and-death issue. Life can be indifferently brutal. This is why it's so important to do everything in your power to avoid as much of this brutality as is humanly possible.

All along, I've been promoting the platform that health is the most important of all human possessions. However, let's be honest, health doesn't motivate people into action until they're dying, and sometimes not even then. Appearance, not health, seems to be one of the few things that inspires people to at least ponder the idea of wanting to lose unwanted body fat. Despite the fact that we are living through an epoch where those employing tortured mental gymnastics are trying to convince the world that we're all beautiful, we're not, and some people are not fooled. Most reasonable people care about their personal appearance. The majority of well-adjusted people don't purposely diminish their outward form. On the rare occasion when a human realistically commits to losing unhealthful body fat, though the commitment may have nothing to do with improving health and everything to do with vanity, at least it's a step in the right direction. Despite this narrow, superficial and ill-advised thought process, an unintended consequence is that health will be served.

It remains to be seen if weight-loss drugs will help our overweight pets. I doubt it insofar as they have, by and large, failed to help their human owners. Over-the-counter weight-loss drugs have failed to stem the tide of rampant over-fat in America. Prescription weight-loss medications barely make a dent. Surgical weight-loss procedures for the morbidly obese won't get the majority down to and keep them at a normal healthful weight for life. Finally, after you read yet another book or article claiming to contain the "sure-fire" secret for weight loss, such as eating based on your blood type, fasting, cleanses, eating no carbs, eating more carbs, eating more protein or maybe it's less protein, or eating anything you want, it might dawn on you that none of these promises are true. Can bariatric surgery in a traditional clinical setting be a future option for over-fat pets? I don't know, but I do think that for pets, as well as their humans, it would be a better idea to simply follow a healthful diet, along with daily exercise.

Big business will not help you, the government will not help you, nor will big-pharma help you. You can hope and pray all you want, but God will not help you either. There are no miracle fixes. Magic is no more than an illusion. Temptation is everywhere. You must learn to deal with these realities or fall by the wayside. Every positive nutritional and fitness-related decision you make is a step in the right direction. If you don't help yourself, your family and your pets, you all become victims waiting to happen. Knowingly placing yourself and those you care about into the role of the victim and then desperately hoping and waiting for someone to be your champion, someone to advocate for your unenviable position, is a losing proposition and only for the pusillanimous among us.

52

Mindset

Nutrition and fitness should be viewed through a singular lens if achieving health is a priority. However, this is not the case because our mindset regarding health has gone so far off the rails. As a result, we find ourselves in a dysfunctional culture with deeply ingrained views that promote defective health. Based on my experiences and observations, I would guess that ninety-some-odd percent of the population adheres to these ingrained views. Our societal evolution has led us to this place. These views are what we desire, what we embrace. These predilections are so pervasive that they are the norm. Normal is the usually accepted condition of being, whether it's right or wrong, whether it's good or bad. Normal is what most people aspire to and ultimately become. Therein lies the problem. We need to change what is considered to be normal if we are ever going to meaningfully improve our health and well-being as a society.

People don't bat an eye at normal. They don't think about it. Normal doesn't engender even the most rudimentary of prehistoric responses. People, simply and unquestioningly, speak about normal things, behave normally and think normally. They "do normal" without giving their actions any critical thought. Normal is what the vast majority is. While I recognize what normal is, I and like-minded people, reject the standard of popular normalcy. People who engage in the health and fitness-positive behaviors I've discussed throughout this book are not normal. They are abnormal by their own definition and most certainly by the definition of normal, which society has deemed acceptable. Despite this abnormal label, they remain grateful for, committed to, and embrace this state of being. Normal behaviors and thinking, especially those concerning health by way of nutrition and fitness, typically lead to unintended, undesirable outcomes. Abnormal behaviors and thought processes alert us to both the blatant and subtle messages being injected into an unenlightened citizenry.

I will illustrate this point for you. On the morning of Thursday, May 27, 2010, I was listening to the news on the radio. These details are very specific because I was so struck by what I heard that I stopped what I was doing to take some notes. I felt they would help me in my work at some time in the future. The radio station was WCBS 880 AM, a New York area all-news station. Every morning at about 4:23 am, radio personality Pat Carroll would do a two-minute or so piece for *Parents Magazine* called "Raising Our Kids," which I found interesting. The broadcasts included a diverse range of topics, such as decorating for the holidays, nutrition for children, health and medical information, and many other issues relevant to parents. On this particular morning, the topic being discussed was about educating our younger kids about food and nutrition, by utilizing the teaching moments that present themselves when we go grocery shopping with our children in tow.

Ms. Carroll was presenting examples of how a parent can play fun yet educational games with kids regarding different kinds of vegetables and fruits. I don't recall all the particulars of the games, but the point was to encourage parents to teach kids about healthful food and proper nutrition in a fun and kid-friendly manner. A couple of examples might include rolling through the produce section and saying to the little one, "I am thinking of a green vegetable whose name begins with the letter B," or "I am thinking of a fruit that is sometimes red whose name begins with the letter A." I'm sure you get the idea. Parents could explain the differences between eating fruit with its naturally occurring sugar and eating processed cereals with their added sugars.

Ms. Carroll did a fine job in submitting a variety of examples that could be utilized by parents during food shopping excursions to educate children about healthful eating, while at the same time engaging and having fun with them. Overall, I thought her ideas were a thoughtful and excellent way to build a foundation for a healthful life at a level commensurate with the age of the kids. Parents must pay more than lip service when it comes to the health of their offspring. They need to take the time and put forth the effort to teach their kids about healthful eating. The adults also need to set a good example. Do as I say, not as I do, will not convince your children of the importance of following a nutritious diet. Will there be bumps in the road? Of course, but this is a poor excuse to acquiesce to the unsound reasoning of a child. It's more important to be a parent than a buddy at this stage. If you are not ready to say "no" to your child, you are not ready for parenthood. If handled with patience, these nutritional education forays into the grocery store will stimulate the kids into critical thinking. They want to please the parents while at the same time demonstrating what they've learned. As a result, simply saying "no" to a child's poor food choices will usually be a last resort.

I believe it's important for kids to be involved in what is being purchased for family meals. This gives them the sense that they are helping in the decision-making process. This is different from asking your kids to pick out the sugary cereal or cookies they want. What I'm suggesting is educating and gently guiding them into sound food decisions while at the same time letting them feel that they arrived at these good decisions on their own. Teaching moments await in every aisle of the food store, even in the processed and junk food aisles.

On balance, the "Raising Our Kids" segment on this day was informative and well done—that is to say, until the end when it became painfully "normal." Had she concluded her piece prior to the last part, I would have tipped my hat to her. Regrettably, Ms. Carroll closed her segment with statements to the effect that parents should save the snack aisle and the "treats" contained therein for last. She indicated that in doing so, parents would then be imparting the lesson that snacks are a sometimes food, not an all-the-time food. At this point, my emotions fluctuated between frustrated, sad resignation at the muted attempts by so-called experts in the health and wellness field to rectify an attitude that's at the root cause of hundreds-of-thousands of preventable illnesses and deaths each year in America alone.

To normal people listening in, the comments regarding snacks and treats voiced at the conclusion of this broadcast wouldn't have induced any more or less of a reaction than any other portion of the report. I'll even go so far as to opine that for most normal listeners, no part of the report stimulated any reaction whatsoever.

It's comments such as these about snacks and treats, and also about other unhealthful foods and beverages that almost subliminally encourage a weak populous, terminally on auto-pilot, to just keep doing the same things over and over again. These comments don't furrow anyone's brow; they're low-key, inoffensive and slip smoothly into our consciousness. Their acceptance and the subsequent behaviors they spawn by an easily manipulated public exemplifies this point. To further exacerbate an already dire situation, we are regularly, blatantly and repeatedly clunked on the head about snack foods, fast foods, junk foods, junk beverages, and all manner of practices which imperil our health—wrapped up and presented in a warm and fuzzy package of Americana or other such emotion inducing claptrap.

We are constantly being managed and herded into specific patterns of behavior. Whether this occurs unobtrusively or boldly, the end result is the same. The vast majority of the population suffers. The message being spewed is that to have fun, to eat the best tasting food, drink the best drinks, be ultra cool and, in many instances—now with the advent of functional foods (food and beverage manufacturers adding vitamins, minerals and other nutrients to otherwise virtually worthless food products)---to improve one's health, one need only surrender as we are gently guided into this mode of thinking by seemingly innocuous reports, purportedly presented for our enlightenment.

Normal is everywhere, from the guy on the news broadcast telling the audience that he can't start his day without a cup of coffee to the talk show host informing us about her needing a drink to unwind at the end of the work day, to the supermarket rags touting their annual holiday heart disease inducing recipes, to the grade school math books posing the problem, "If John has 5 candy bars and gives 2 away, how many candy bars does John have left?" Why not apples? Why not bananas? Why not use some healthful piece of fruit or a vegetable? Why are the majority of the examples in these math and reading books junk food? Because it's all normal. We are buried under an avalanche of toxic normalcy. It's all we see and all we hear. We are seeing with our eyes and hearing with our ears, but there seems to be a disconnect before the information reaches the supercomputer, which is our brain, preventing us from engaging with it in a thoughtful, reasonable and logical manner.

This is the general mindset of an America that has obliviously bought into this type of thinking, including regarding snacks as treats and treats as snacks. Goodies, special occasion foods and drinks, sometimes foods, sinful indulgences, comfort food, tasty delights, sweets, fun foods, party foods and drinks, bar grub, and a host of other seemingly benign sobriquets have lulled the masses into a nutritional torpor. All of these "treats" and the attitude that embraces their consumption, along with other injurious behaviors, are the reasons why most of America is copiously fed yet undernourished, unfit, over-fat, sickly, overmedicated, prematurely aging, whiny, and an excuse-making mess.

Parents Magazine, by way of Ms. Carroll's "Raising Our Kids" report, and WCBS 880 AM would have taken a bold step in the right direction toward addressing the abysmal state of American nutrition in general and childhood nutrition specifically, had they treated the subject with the unwavering attitude it deserves. How about giving our kids a fighting chance at a healthy life by telling them the unvarnished truth about the garbage contained in the snack food aisles of supermarkets? How about educating children about the dangers and potential hazards of consuming that garbage? How about informing the kids that most of the items, loosely referred to as food, sold in grocery stores are unacceptable to those who cherish their health?

Living, breathing examples abound in supermarkets, and especially in snack food aisles, painfully depicting the ramifications of poor food choices. Tell your kids to look around at the rest of the shoppers reaching for those tasty treats. People who, through no fault other than their own dreadful choices, waddle to grab that box of cookies, candy, snack cakes and junk cereal. Tell your kids to look at the physical condition of the overwhelming number of shoppers loading up on chips, soda, doughnuts, ice cream and junk peanut butter. Point out to the children how these people have allowed trash food to transform them into overweight, minimally ambulatory versions of their former selves. Make them take notice of the over-fat people whose posteriors hang over to encompass the seats of the motorized shopping carts upon which they ride. Indicate to the youngsters how some of these riders don't even bother to get off of their motorized shopping carts to grab their goodies, treats and snacks. The effort would apparently be too great. Instead, they employ the use of gripping tongs to reach out and grasp these delights.

In addition to the effort they would need to generate to actually get up and out of their conveyance and locomote to the shelf to reach for the item, many of these folks are tethered to oxygen tanks via a clear plastic hose hooked under their nose. It's too much of a hassle to do much of anything once you've reduced your life to this sad state. Yet, here they are, in the aisle of treats. And how are those treats treating them? Explain to kids the tremendous and totally avoidable health risks that come with consuming these products and adhering to a way of life that, in fact, encourages their consumption.

Indeed, educate your kids at the supermarket. Make them aware that more than 7 out of 10 members of our population are over-fat. Don't neglect to explain to the youngsters that just because the others are skinny doesn't make them healthy. Point out how most of these people arrived at this abysmal state of being. Teach them to be compassionate toward those who are genetically, biologically and medically over-fat, but not to accept any of these legitimate reasons as a convenient excuse when easily avoidable self-destructive behaviors are the cause. Illustrate how the media and our sick culture at large attempt to paint all over-fat, unfit people as victims, conveniently conflating those who are in the minority and afflicted through no fault of their own with those who have no one to blame other than themselves. Point out how victimhood is always highlighted while personal responsibility receives nary a passing nod.

Tell your children how all the heavily marketed garbage food, laced with ingredients to ensure their delicious tastes, played the pivotal role in the decimation of the health of most of these sorry souls. Prompt them to take a good look around while informing them that if they don't make the right choices, they're looking directly into the face of their future. If you really care about your children, if you want them to develop into intelligent, responsible adults who realize the worthiness of being as healthy and fit as possible, then, and only then, will you teach them excellent alternatives to mass-produced trash food. Then, and only then, will you tell them that normal treats, snacks, cereals, drinks and fast foods are not sometimes foods but never foods.

Educate them on the concept that there's no room for moderation when it comes to their health, then follow through at home. Set a good example by what you purchase and eat. Your children look up to you. You run the show. Do not cave into the whimsical demands of children who lack the cognitive ability of adults and are easily manipulated by advertisers and peer pressure. As a parent, you are the primary educator. Take on this role with the gravity it deserves. You didn't bring children into this world to sicken them, kill them or contribute more fools to a population already burgeoning with fools.

Tell them that if they don't agree with you, they'll be free one day to make their own food choices. At least they'll be able to make those choices armed with honest information, not mindless drivel. If they go on to make poor choices when they are no longer in your charge, that's on them. They can't claim ignorance. As a parent, you can't do any more than this.

I sometimes ponder the constant, indulgent behaviors attributable to normal people regarding treats and snacks. To my way of thinking, if the normal population considers item "X" a treat, what does this imply about the rest of the things they eat? That their food choices are not tasty enough? As far as I'm concerned, these individuals consume unhealthful fats, sodium and sugar in just about everything they eat. It's all tasty. One would think they were being force-fed a steady diet of some awful flavored swill most of the time while being treated to something deliciously infused with fat, sodium and sugar only on special occasions. Normal people already have a putrid diet teeming with all three of these ingredients, not to mention the chemical additives. This toxic witch's brew of ingredients certainly and undeniably provides a tempting flavor-fest. How much more "treating themselves" do these people require?

When you know how to eat, everything is a treat. Nothing is better than anything else, just different. When you learn how to enjoy preparing and eating healthful foods, there's no need to wait for sinful indulgences because everything you eat tastes great and has the added benefit of being healthful. In this case, there are no sins. Looking forward to every meal, from a health perspective as well as a taste perspective, becomes the rule rather than the exception. There is no need to compromise. In this situation, even your deserts are packed with nutrients and are considered meals instead of empty gratifications serving no purpose other than to satisfy a want.

Of course, for the best results you must commit to a different way of life other than the one to which you are accustomed. There is no getting around the irrefutable fact that desire alone is insufficient in order to attain your overall wellness goals and more specific nutritional goals. Discipline, determination and preparedness to say no to your detrimental behaviors are essential. You must educate yourself in order to learn and progress. Any fool can make rubbish palatable by adding the normal cooking ingredients—salt, sugar and fat. Doing so does a complete disservice to your taste buds, to say nothing of your health and that of your family.

Once you've acquired the knowledge required to cook and eat healthfully, your health will begin to improve. Instead of robotically reaching for the normal cooking ingredients mentioned above, regular use of herbs and spices to season food will become the norm. At first, your food may taste bland. In a few weeks or so, your taste buds will come back to life. You'll actually taste your food instead of tasting only salt, sugar and fat. When you reach this point, even minimal saltiness or sweetness in food will be pronounced. Remember, rejecting the normal American diet and replacing it with wholesome foods is akin to a drug addict going through detox after quitting drugs. It's hard work, but the rewards are well worth the effort.

My purpose for writing this book was not to provide you with recipes. Perhaps one day I'll write a cookbook, but this is definitely not it. This work is intended to be a cautionary message, in essence, a warning I suggest you heed before it's too late. This one is an attempt to get you to open your eyes, ears and ultimately your mind as to how you are being played by a flawed cultural system. For the benefit of you and your family, you must be aware that average people are kept in a state of normalcy and herded like cattle by other, more powerful people who have agendas. Their agendas have nothing to do with keeping you and yours healthy but a lot to do with keeping their pockets full of your money.

Further, it should anger you, as it does me, when the many powers that comprise society, obfuscate, out-and-out lie, sugar-coat, manipulate or treat the citizenry as if we were all imbeciles. I respect naked, unvarnished reality. I believe in receiving the truth no matter how painful. As such, I also deliver my messages in this manner and then leave the receivers of these messages alone to do whatever they desire with the information provided. I would much rather have you disagree with me based on sound, personal reasoning as a result of what I convey to you about nutrition and fitness in our culture. Good, reliable, common-sense information is hard to come by. I find it tiresome and unacceptable to entertain arguments based on the "party line."

We live in an age where a tremendous amount of information is readily available and instantly attainable. Information about nutrition, fitness and overall health is no exception. There are very few legitimate excuses for not being aware of the most rudimentary, beneficial health practices. The problem is not the unavailability of positive wellness directions but the failure by those individuals who have the facts to implement them. Once you have received good information, if you still have a burning desire to remain part of the herd, that's up to you. Do I have an opinion if you make this choice? Absolutely, and it's pretty obvious because of what I've written in this book. But who cares? We all live as we wish. Regrettably, we don't all die as we would prefer. No matter what anyone decides, it won't change what I do every day—exercise and eat healthful food. I'll also continue to shrug off, as fools, those who know better yet insist on traveling down the same dysfunctional, illogical path, only to complain about their woeful health outcomes, nonetheless.

Useless words are the partners of useless behaviors. From politicians to newscasters and everyone in between, normal people are fond of making hollow statements. They find nothing wrong with the content of their words because these meaningless utterances are socially accepted by a predominantly tone-deaf population. In short, it is another example of the prevailing normal mindset in our culture and society at large. This mindset continues to promote and contribute to the deterioration of our health. It also makes people sound like buffoons.

For example, some years ago, an acquaintance of mine died as a result of a heart attack. He was a pleasant enough fellow, barely 50 years old, overweight, a non-exerciser, a drinker, smoker and ate the type of food that just about everyone eats. He was doing what most people refer to as "living." He was obviously treating himself, using the socially accepted definition of the word. By society's standards, a very normal guy.

As news of this unfortunate individual's death began to circulate among his colleagues, friends and acquaintances, they all, at least as I was able to discern, expressed sorrow and shock. I was able to comprehend their sorrow, and I shared this feeling. As I stated, he was pleasant. Predictably, people began making the usual inane statements, the most popular being, "I'm shocked and can't believe he's gone." Shock? Based on his lifestyle, I was shocked, not by the fact that he died of a heart attack, but by the fact that he hadn't died of one sooner. Of course, when some of our mutual acquaintances brought up the subject, and I expressed this opinion, I was quickly labeled an insensitive asshole. Most people are blinded to reality by society's ritualistic niceties. The commonly paid price for insisting to dwell in this realm of delusion is often one's life. We are expected to express shock when someone dies. It's considered the right thing to do. American culture has a very uncomfortable relationship with death. It's as if the general idea is that death is something that happens to other people, particularly old people. There is some sort of automatic defense mechanism—which is actually a self-destruct mechanism—built into people's psyche that proclaims, "Don't worry, eat and drink with gusto, enjoy life to the fullest." There is nothing built in that instructs us to think critically. This must be taught, learned and applied. Hopefully, this occurs before we kill ourselves by making really bad choices.

I would not have been shocked (saddened, yes) if a healthy person who ate what I consider to be a proper diet, worked out and didn't drink or smoke suddenly died of a heart attack. No one gets to live forever despite our best efforts. We all die, everyone: the elderly, the young, the sick, as well as the healthy. It's part of the experience. Being shocked by the death of someone who is obviously committing slow suicide plainly illustrates just how unaccepting our culture is of harsh reality, and this is to our overall detriment. As I've mentioned, we have no guarantees, no matter how we live. The best we can do is to improve our odds. If we do this, we can do no more.

Don't be shocked when an unfit, overweight, self-indulgent individual dies. When all the normal people are asking, "Can you believe he's dead?" the only possible answer that makes any rational sense is, "Yes, I most certainly can believe he's dead." This is another teaching opportunity for you and a learning moment for your kids. Inform the young that a substantial number of people who live a certain way die as a result of their chosen way of living. No shock here, just unvarnished reality.

When you begin to take notice of unthinkingly accepted and embraced normal occurrences, and they resonate as infuriatingly absurd, such as radio personalities making comments as I described earlier, or people practicing pointless, ritualistic conformities for the sake of appearing socially correct, as when expressing utter shock at the death of someone who was obviously killing himself, when you start to notice these things, then you are on your way to a logical perspective. Do not accept the ridiculous. So many of the ingrained behaviors that go unchallenged in our culture directly and indirectly contribute to our declining health, the degradation of the environment, and threaten the overall wellness of humans as a species. You should be angry and generate this anger into positive health-promoting actions for you and your family. Or, you can insist on acting like a stupid cow, in a single file, following along with the rest of the stupid cows, marching blithely into the bolt gun. Just don't express last-second shock when you realize what's about to happen.

There exist an innumerable amount of normal behaviors and attitudes. Some are neutral, some have benefits, and a large number continue to cause harm. It seems that in America today, when the discussion turns toward nutrition, fitness and general health, the normal state of being for most is one of mental illness, which usually leads to a premature death.

Teach your children to listen and to critically observe their surroundings. Make them aware of the seemingly innocuous cultural happenings which serve to groom them for maintaining the status quo; a status quo that encourages and perpetuates detrimental health practices. Most adults, let alone children, are oblivious. They're far too busy watching reality TV and counting their "likes" on social media. If adults choose to kill themselves as a result of poor lifestyle choices, they should at least embark on their suicide-by-food missions after a blunt, no-nonsense briefing concerning the odds of their surviving said mission. Flirting with disastrous health outcomes should only be attempted voluntarily. Reckless, impetuous souls should not be manipulated nor inveigled into risking their health and, more than likely, their lives.

As far as your kids are concerned, they should not be allowed the option of death by food and "fitness-less." Like adults, children need to be educated and provided with straightforward, candid information. We must stop finding words and reasons which guiltlessly give us a pass on stupid health behaviors, and must instead seek out words and reasons demonstrating why stupid health behaviors need to be eliminated. We are all being assaulted by propaganda, misinformation, healthwashing (greenwashing's equally evil sibling), peer pressure and feeble, watered-down nutritional advice. It's plain to see that adults have eaten the bait (literally as well as figuratively).

That being the case, if we don't experience a cultural epiphany, what chance do children, being more susceptible to exploitation than their parents, have of growing up without preventable diseases? Only a gambler's chance and this is unacceptable. Having been armed with good information as children, adults can make their own choices based on that good information. If they make poor choices for themselves, these choices will not be the result of a lack of knowledge, just different priorities. The time is long overdue for kids to be dealt with in an honest fashion. It is said that they are tomorrow's leaders. As such, they are our only hope for a healthful future. America needs to readjust its mindset.

53
Sensitivity Police

As is usually the case with the implementation of most seemingly reasonable ideas, unintended consequences arise. It was no different when small, prehistoric social groups began to coalesce into much larger societies in an attempt to benefit the greater good. However, despite all the warm and fuzzy talk about people being social creatures, human nature prohibits us from being the quintessential social beings many imagine or would like us to be. The reality is that we can only take our fellow human beings for so long. Too many divergent opinions, agendas and sensibilities among ourselves are guaranteed to cause friction at some point, which in turn erupts into a full-blown flame of vitriol and hostility.

As a baby boomer, I've lived through some pretty tumultuous times. By way of example, the 1960s were something to behold, encompassing civil rights struggles, assassinations of prominent national leaders, the Vietnam War, college campus unrest and race riots, which overwhelmed major U.S. cities. I don't know if it's because the world is so much better connected, allowing more news to circulate almost instantly, but writing this now, I feel the present is more explosive than the 1960s. In the last generation or so, a slew of issues could no longer be contained and burst their societal seams. One social problem melds into the next as they overlap one another. There seems to be no end.

Oppressed peoples in various nations erupting in protest and violence against their totalitarian leaders, school and mass shootings, festering racism and ethnic prejudice, veterans' concerns, religious fanaticism, domestic and international terrorism, obscene healthcare costs, homelessness, climate change, women's rights, immigration issues, fair pay for workers, education problems, the general toxification and degradation of the environment, cyber attacks against critical infrastructure, food insecurity, abuse of children by those to whom our children are entrusted, ageism, challenges facing the intellectually and physically disabled, animal welfare, inequality in taxation, big corporate money in politics, partisan politics and the aftermath of the COVID-19 pandemic, with not only its obvious negative health consequences, but also with the societal divisiveness it caused, are but some of the issues plaguing us at present, and I've only scratched the surface.

As a result of societal upheaval, attitudes are constantly changing, as does the language we use to convey these new attitudes. We are living in a time where sensitivity in both perspective and expression has pushed back strongly against inconsiderate beliefs and words from bygone days. The term "political correctness" is a direct result of these changes. Many of these cultural transformations and current points of view are welcome and long overdue. However, as is always the wont of so many human beings, things are taken too far, become ridiculous and often detrimental to our welfare.

The recent overemphasis on a sensitive, non-threatening, inoffensive approach to nutrition, fitness and overall wellness is a clear example of things having gone awry. It's just not working. There never was, and will probably never exist, given human nature, a balance between societal entities promoting all manner of unhealthful behaviors and those seeking to save humanity from itself. Those tempting and pushing us to behave in ways that promote illness and death by far outnumber those trying to sound the alarm that we are killing ourselves. Let's face it: commercials and advertisements for fast-food and beer far out number the push to consume more fruits and vegetables.

As if the inequity between common sense and succumbing to tasty self-destruction were not enough, along come the sensitivity police and the body-positivity promoters. These people are so intent on rectifying real and perceived injustices that they utilize hyperbolic, feel-good rhetoric to further their agenda. They attempt to marginalize and make irrelevant anyone not embracing their type of jargon. They liberally take offense to any criticism that goes counter to their agenda. They tell us that everyone is beautiful. The reality is they are guilty of fusing different issues in an effort to get society to see it their way. A person can be physically ugly as sin, yet have a beautiful character, soul, personality, essence or heart; call it what you will. On the other hand, a morally corrupt, rotten-to-the-core, evil, diabolical monster can be housed in a physically attractive body. We need to be very careful and quite specific about what we're talking about when we paint people with such broad brush strokes. If my words offend you, tough, because I'm offended at your being offended. Turnabout is fair play.

It is said that beauty is subjective and exists in the eye of the beholder, or, more bluntly, there is a toilet seat for every ass. I generally agree. However, as much as many humans need to see themselves apart from the animal kingdom, we are, indeed, animals. As with animals of the non-human variety, the furtherance of the species depends on attracting a mate. As such, even though the sensitivity police/body positivity crusaders are loath to acknowledge this reality, there exists for all creatures, humans included, a general standard of beauty and attraction. Survival of the fittest depends on this.

Where humans are concerned, there is quite a bit of latitude; therefore, we have different classifications for different body types. Mesomorph refers to a naturally muscular body type. Endomorphs naturally carry a higher amount of body fat and are rounder, but not necessarily obese. Ectomorphs are naturally thin, with small joints and long, lean limbs. A person can fall into any of these categories, all of which are obviously diverse, and still be fit and healthy. A person can also be a combination of any of these categories and be fit and healthy. It's when we start coloring beyond the rough parameters of these physical standards that we encourage entirely preventable health problems.

It is nothing more than wishful thinking and propaganda to say that everyone is physically beautiful. It does a disservice to those struggling with the self-induced diseases of Western society. It creates a loophole and provides an easy escape hatch for people who will rely on the false narrative that they are beautiful. It fails to educate and promotes an attitude that you can eat and drink anything you like, and the consequences of disease be damned. It provides no motivation to improve. It sends a deadly message to our children. It sets up the next and ensuing generations for the same illnesses and resultant preventable deaths as all the previous generations.

The "everyone is beautiful" mantra sounds nice, but it's dangerous and reserved for blind, unrealistic fools. You may be a very nice person, but when I look at you I see a person living in a poorly maintained house, just waiting for it to collapse. Dogmatically espousing and blindly following the credo that "everyone is beautiful" completely ignores the millions of "beautiful" people with heart disease, certain cancers, elevated serum cholesterol, diabetes and all the other diseases caused by their "beauty." Sure, everyone's beautiful until they're not.

54

Cost To Healthcare

The cost for healthcare in America is astronomical. The United States spends more money on healthcare than any other country on the planet, yet it is comfortably nestled in rank among those countries with the most dismal healthcare outcomes. This has become common knowledge and would be a glaring embarrassment to our elected officials were it not for their seeming immunity to such pedestrian emotions. I won't bore you with the tedious numbers because most people don't care, that is until they become sick and have to pay for medications, medical procedures and hospital stays. The numerous publications of these costs have done nothing to change the suicidal health habits of the population. Suffice to say, these monumental costs continue to crush us, as well as what is referred to as our healthcare system, which I touched upon earlier as nothing more than our disease maintenance system.

We have been in the midst of a public health crisis for decades, which is killing hundreds of thousands of citizens every year. Despite this, very few, and certainly not elected officials, policy makers or politicians, take the situation seriously. A killer virus has panache, but people dropping dead as a result of preventable diseases caused by poor eating and exercise habits is not a sexy or dramatic enough issue to get behind. This is especially true when you consider that most of the people who are in a position to sound the alarm are themselves guilty of questionable eating, drinking and exercise behaviors. These very same individuals periodically make some noise about the dangers of obesity, but obesity is just one part of a much bigger health problem.

Government officials and other authorities are very good at making themselves appear to be on top of an issue that, for one reason or another, gains some popular traction. Obesity is one such issue. However, do we really need more bipartisan committees, studies, Senate subcommittees, think tanks, investigative committees and pontification on the subject before we implement meaningful policies and remedial actions required to stop and reverse our nose-dive into food-induced narcosis? It's all been done; talk and more talk. That's where leadership excels—in talking. If we continue with our current attitudes and behaviors about health and fitness, the United States of America, our country's proud name, will become meaningless, no more than a barren retrospective of dignity long ago evaporated.

Most of the solutions proposed by those who are purportedly concerned with the well-being of Americans and rising healthcare costs, whose ascension into the stratosphere shows no sign of diminishing and which can be easily linked to poor personal choices, do no more than scratch the surface of the problem. These suggested fixes in the form of programs, initiatives, campaigns and the like, proclaimed to the citizenry through catchy names and trendy, witty slogans, further enhanced through the promotion of pins, ribbons, wristbands and other such folderols, will not get the job done. The job will not get done in this manner because, in this country, we don't have a majority with the desire or will to do what it takes to fix the state of our abysmal health. Eradication of our disease maintenance mentality, which is the foundation of our exorbitant health costs, is required. We are much more interested in symbolism than substance. Our woeful state of all things health-related is exacerbated because we are a society that worships all things skinny, but our societal bipolar disorder is always in full bloom as we incessantly promote and engage in asinine eating and drinking. For the most part, these behaviors cause us to pack on unhealthful excess fat. We are the dumbest, laziest, excuse-making, non-responsibility-taking, fattest, skinny-worshipping people around.

Years ago policy makers in some locales passed legislation requiring restaurants and certain retail establishments to post calorie content on their menus and provide nutritional information upon request. This was done in an effort to educate the public and provide transparency in the hope that such information would assist people in making better food choices. A similar logic was used on defined packaged foods of some manufacturers. It would stand to reason that a better-informed public, making better food choices, would lead to a less disease-riddled public, eventually cutting healthcare costs. Since I believe in providing the people with honest information, these ideas appeal to me. They were a step in the right direction toward nutritional sanity; a small step long in coming, but a positive one, nonetheless.

However, I further believe that all restaurants and food makers should openly provide nutrition and ingredient information on packaging and menus without exception, not just fast-food establishments. Expensive, exclusive restaurants requiring three months advance reservations also serve their share of artery-clogging, heart disease-inducing meals. In this sense, they are no better than run-of-the-mill diners, fast-food joints and chain restaurants serving greasy, deep-fried bar fare. The only difference is that you get to contribute to your own demise in pretentious surroundings while enjoying the privilege of paying extortionate prices.

In an effort to supposedly save people from themselves, the federal government, albeit with the expected loopholes, banned trans fats a few years ago. Many local governments are considering a tax on sugary beverages, which has created conflicts between them and state governments, who frown upon the locals taxing soda and other sugary drinks. Efforts by governments to ban problematic food, drink and the like have been criticized by some as an attempt by the government to enact a "nanny state."

Sadly, incongruous agendas and incompatible priorities between influential people in both the public and private sectors prevent, or at best hamper, the efforts of government officials desiring to promote more healthful plans, no matter how inadequate they are, to pass laws. The health of the population with its associated numbing and societally ponderous healthcare costs are obviously not primary concerns for everyone.

While I have strong feelings about lowering healthcare costs in America by improving the health of its people, I'm ambivalent about the government becoming overly involved because I don't trust its purity of intent. We always walk a precarious path when we require governmental assistance since its history of intervention is replete with unintended consequences and, regrettably, purposeful missteps that defy logic. Generally, the government is in too much of our business as things stand. Over one-hundred years ago, the constitutional ban on the production, sale and importation, but not consumption of, alcoholic beverages during the Prohibition Era failed miserably.

Largely influenced by religious groups, much earlier attempts in America by temperance organizations to reduce and abstentionists to banish alcoholic beverages also ultimately ended in failure. Alcohol and tobacco products are directly and indirectly responsible for untold disease and death. Today, while there are prohibitive age restrictions in place to limit their sale to younger people, these harmful products are not banned. There are plenty of toxic ingredients contained within products we use on a daily basis to which most people pay no mind, including many of those people whose job it is to protect the public welfare, our elected officials. What governments permit and what they ban seems arbitrary to me, and I mostly don't trust their judgement on these matters due to their own biases and the undue influence of corporate America upon their decisions.

While I contend that it remains a positive step toward transparency, nutrition and ingredient information on packaging and menus will not prevent people from eating fast food and highly processed foods or suddenly make them health conscious. Do you really believe that the movers and shakers in our decadent and self-indulgent society are going to stop dining at upscale restaurants because they are provided with information alerting them to the potential health hazards of what they are stuffing themselves with? All this information will not do enough to turn the tide of people killing themselves with food.

Most people are over-fat, unfit and too busy eating or thinking about eating unhealthful food to think about being health conscious. They gorge on this stuff because it's fatty, salty, sweet and tastes good. It's too much of an effort for them to cook because convenience trumps health almost every time, and unhealthful food is relatively inexpensive. If they can afford expensive, fancy, unhealthful food, so much the better. Follow the simple logic. Let's stop complicating the issue and making excuses for everyone. For most, health, fitness and nutritional concerns dwell in that portion of the brain reserved for other distasteful topics such as death and taxes. We know it's important to face these issues, but we are not trained to do so. In extreme cases, despite a medical crisis, some folks still refuse to change their behaviors.

I find it interesting when someone literally kills him or herself through health negligence and indifference, and friends and family display shock at this death. They inevitably discount the facts that the individual was 50 pounds over-fat, on blood pressure, cholesterol and diabetes medication, exercised sporadically and ate the typical garbage most people eat. We always hear the same moronic comments about the deceased, such as, "He seemed to be managing all his illnesses with his medications. He took them religiously. He walked on the treadmill for an hour. He went for annual physicals, and generally, his numbers were good. I just saw him yesterday. This is such a shock." Spare me the trite wake whisperings. It's not a shock when a person such as this dies. The person I've just described is a typical citizen, just like the millions of others in America who have fooled themselves into believing you can have it both ways. You cannot.

More surprising is when a person who consistently exercised, as I've prescribed throughout, ate the right things for the right reasons, completely avoided what the masses refer to as treats, and avoided all the socially acceptable crutches including, but not limited to, alcoholic beverages and smoking—when this type of individual suddenly dies, then that my friend is a shock. Nevertheless, this kind of person was dedicated to the most healthful way of life personally attainable. In his last moments, he wouldn't have been questioning or lamenting, having made poor health choices. He did his best. One can ask for nothing more. Sometimes shit happens that is completely beyond our ability to control. We can't worry about that.

People either care about their health or they don't. Governments either care about their healthcare systems or they don't. It's black and white in both instances. Caring about health and the system we depend on to support it, just a little, or moderately, is tantamount to being a little or moderately pregnant. Walking on a treadmill for an hour, even daily, doesn't necessarily make one healthy. It certainly does very little for you if you are simply strolling and not focused on reasonably challenging yourself on the machine. Further, if you are managing your illnesses, as is so popular today, with various medications, remaining over-fat, but continue to make dreadful food and drink choices, you can walk from here to Mumbai, and it won't matter. What people such as these want is to continue indulging in their self-destructive behaviors, go for a physical and pray for a thumbs-up from the doctor. Even if they get a thumbs-up, so what? It's virtually meaningless. Maybe not today or tomorrow, but certainly one day for most, this unhealthful yet typical manner of living takes its toll. Sometimes, you just drop dead.

Based on decades of discussions concerning nutrition, fitness and overall health in general, I've come to the conclusion that most people are more ignorant about this particular subject group than even I thought possible. Still, I would like to believe that these same people have at least a rudimentary grasp of what constitutes healthful and unhealthful behaviors. Whether they engage in it or not, the rich, as well as the poor know exercise to be a necessary habit for health. They know that typical fast food and ultra-processed foods, junk food by any other name, are extremely unhealthful. I would expect that they realize that even consuming too much healthful food will cause them to become over-fat. Maybe I'm giving them too much credit.

In every sector of society, I contend that the astronomical costs to American healthcare, and no doubt to the healthcare of other nations, is directly and indirectly attributable to this low level of fitness and nutrition knowledge. Combine an elementary interpretation of this critical, life-saving subject matter with a lack of meaningful leadership from our elected officials, which in turn fosters an environment of apathy and indifference throughout the land, further diminishing the grave importance of nutrition and fitness; it's no wonder that America is the land of the over-fed, over-fat, undernourished, unfit, over-medicated, and of those paying more for healthcare than in any other place on the planet.

As I stated, adding nutrition and ingredient information describing what you're about to eat to packages and menus is a start, but it's a drop in the ocean. We desperately need so much more in order to have a significant, positive health impact on our citizens. If we are going to be realistic about drastically reducing the cost of healthcare in America, dramatic and sweeping changes are the only solution. Healthcare costs become less, if more people are healthy. I'm aware that this statement doesn't completely eradicate the healthcare cost problem. Nevertheless, getting the majority of the population healthy would make a huge difference.

Of course, we'd need to address the other reasons for our broken healthcare system in order for it to improve. People should be angry and ashamed that they permit a culture that fosters self-destructive behavior to continue, mostly unabated. Something radically different needs to be done to rein in drug costs, the cost of medical procedures and health insurance so that all people can afford them, not just the rich. Ponderous bureaucracies, unscrupulous pharmaceutical companies and middle-men have placed their profits ahead of the general welfare of the people for far too long. Doctors over-prescribing unnecessary medications and procedures and knowing little about nutrition, while being reluctant to tell patients to drop body fat, contribute to rocketing healthcare costs. Doctors, nurses and other healthcare workers need to take a long, hard look in the mirror. Most are less than inspiring, to say the least, as it is blatantly apparent that they are little concerned in leading a healthful life. Medical and nursing schools need to do a much better job of training their students in the areas of disease prevention through nutrition and fitness. Most medical professionals lack the tools and convictions to dispense good advice concerning this matter; therefore, they have little credibility. All of these issues, great and small, contribute in some way to paying more for healthcare.

The fact that healthcare itself is big business gives me a creepy feeling. What is the prime directive of big business, or any business for that matter? Of course, to make money, to profit. Doesn't the thought of "for-profit" hospitals and these "for-profit" healthcare groups that seem to be popping up in so many towns give you pause? Yes, accidents and trauma will always keep medical establishments, health insurance companies and drug makers in the black, but a steady, dependable stream of medically managed folks whose various maladies are self-induced and encouraged by society, now that's a big money maker! Sick people are walking (and sometimes not) dollar signs. Does the healthcare system really want everyone to be healthy? Rhetorical question.

Throughout, I've described the reasons, as I see them, why most of our population, and as a result, the healthcare system itself, are both sick. How do we fix this? For starters, we need an integrative approach. There is no exclusive measure that will resolve the issues of a broken healthcare system caused by a mostly indifferent nation suffering the self-inflicted ravages of being over-fat and unfit. As I mentioned paragraphs ago, nutrition labeling standards are a beginning. We also need restrictions on food marketing. We're always conducting studies on one thing or another. Someone should do a study on the percentage of garbage food advertising versus ads for vegetables, fruits, whole grains, beans, nuts, seeds and legumes. To be clear, I'm not referring to those healthful foods rendered inferior by the usual additives. However, it should be quite evident to even the most unobservant, unaware individual that disease-inducing foods win in a landslide.

Marketing fast food, processed food, junk food, sugary cereals and sugary/salty snack foods to children needs to end. These companies are selling disease. At the very least, we need balance. We need to see just as many, if not more, ads for healthful fare. If the producers of healthful foods don't have the advertising dollars to compete with the multi-billion dollar purveyors of disease-promoting foods, then governments should do what they were elected to do: protect the people and step in with powerful public service announcements each time and right after an ad is aired trying to seduce us or our children into eating and drinking something we will ultimately regret. The only way to make the public aware of what's going on is to keep repeating it, just as good parents do with their children.

When it sees fit, the government levies taxes. Just as taxes were imposed and raised on cigarettes, an absolutely unnecessary and deadly product which sane society would be much better off without, so should they be imposed on all the unnecessary food and drink I've described throughout. I don't like the general idea of governments banning things. We have too many laws and regulations as it stands. Adults should have the right to eat and drink what they want. However, if one wishes to make poor nutritional choices, choices which go counter to all that has been proven and become known to most people about what constitutes a healthful diet, then they should pay for the luxury of slowly killing themselves. The extra tax dollars could be used to fund the government's public service campaign for nutrition and to lower health insurance premiums for those who guard their precious health, but not for those who squander it. As you can see, healthcare costs can also be used as an incentive to lower healthcare costs. Good behavior should be rewarded, whereas bad behavior should be discouraged. To those who won't change, fine, but I don't want to pay for your stupid behaviors. Pay for them yourselves.

Besides taxing us to death, the government is also fond of subsidies. Instead of, by way of example, continuing to subsidize the fossil fuel industry, which encourages their use and results in

250

and contributes to the unintended negative consequences we are all too familiar with—from climate change to catastrophic oil spills, the government should subsidize and promote organic farming, including organic hydroponic farming in neglected and blighted urban neighborhood spaces. This could lead to the development of nutrition and fitness education workshops in these same buildings for area residents. The citizens could be taught to grow food and eventually be provided with employment opportunities at these very same facilities. Teaching people how to eat properly and providing jobs at the same time is a win-win situation. Sometimes, a small thing leads to a positive domino effect. Think what could be accomplished with many, many small things!

Public awareness begins with education. Education should begin at home, but what is usually taught at home regarding nutrition and fitness is sorely lacking, to say the least. That leaves it up to the school system. Sadly, the nutrition and fitness education occurring in school systems doesn't appear to be much better than those lessons being taught at home. States need to implement quality nutrition, cooking and physical education curricula in grades K-12. Nothing against other subjects because I believe in learning, and I'm interested in all manner of topics. Nonetheless, I believe that in the long run, it's, if not more important, at the very least just as important, to know how to feed oneself properly in order to avoid disease, premature death, and ultimately live a long, productive, independent life. Forced to choose, I'd prefer the nutritional/fitness information over another history lesson, which humans seldom learn from anyway, as they continue to make the same mistakes. Further, if schools are for learning and the training of a critically thinking, knowledgeable citizenry, let's immediately stop utilizing schools as indoctrinating boot camps for our children into a culture of lousy food habits. If we're going to teach proper nutrition, we must begin by eliminating in-class parties where junk food is available.

Despite all the talk about improving school food, that's what it amounts to in most school districts, again—talk. We sure are one loquacious society! If you don't believe me, do an online search of school menus throughout our country. The menus remain appalling, in defiance of all the political bluster we hear about improving school meals. Adding an apple or random vegetable to a menu that still contains and considers such health abominations as Kellogg's Pop-Tarts and Nutri-Grain Cereal Bars, Quaker Strawberry Crisp Bars, General Mills Fruity Cheerios and Doritos Nacho Cheese Chips to be part of a nutritious, well-balanced meal plan, is not what any thinking human would recognize as an improvement to school food, unless, that is, one wishes to engage in semantics. Schools need to eliminate all ultra-processed, sugary, salty, oily, chemically infused foods. Junk food vending machines have got to go, as do soda, energy drinks and all soft drink vending machines. We need to make health the priority here. Without health, nothing else matters. Without health, all that remain are sickness and death.

Another strategy that can be used to improve America's health and lessen the burden on her healthcare system is for the government to incentivize producers and sellers of healthful foods to set up shop in low-income and underserved neighborhoods. These areas would include poor urban, as well as, poor rural communities. Incentives could be in the form of tax breaks for retailers, regulatory modifications, lower construction cost deals for the building of new food stores, grants, deferred and/or lower property tax breaks for retailers committed to serving the community's health and wellness with real food. This same strategy could be used to further develop, improve and expand every aspect of the healthful food supply chain from farm to plate. What's needed are commitment, imagination and cooperation.

I've already made it evident that I'm no big fan of the government getting any more involved in our lives than is absolutely necessary. Still, it would be naive of me to believe that our healthcare and the nation's health in general would not be improved without some assistance from those in charge. Governmental regulatory agencies, as a matter of course, prohibit certain additives to a wide variety of products we routinely use. This is because these additives pose a danger to human health and, therefore, are not recognized as safe for certain uses, including, but not limited to, ingestion and topical application. If those in authority would embrace this same logic where our food is concerned and finally come to terms with the irrefutable fact that ultra-processed junk-food and fast food are contributing to disease and death due to additives such as sugar, salt, oils and innumerable chemicals, essentially creating palatable, non-nutritious pseudo-foods, and banned the addition of these nutritionally gratuitous ingredients, they would be doing a great service to the citizenry. We need to improve the quality of our food, particularly convenience foods. These products are in need of reformulation if we're serious about the health of the country.

55

Childhood Obesity/Overweight

America is a nation of mostly fat people who are getting fatter. If I were exploring over-fat from a strictly aesthetic perspective, I'd say, so what? To each his own. Beauty is in the eye of the beholder, as the saying goes. In that case, I would have no need to write this book. However, and despite the fact that we humans, as I've already mentioned, are conceived in such a way that we fall into the three general categories of ectomorph, endomorph and mesomorph, I am not strictly discussing aesthetics. In recent years, positive cultural shifts have occurred, causing attitudes to change about the way we treat one another. There is a palpable mainstream movement afoot which seeks to end bullying, shaming, inequality and basic insensitivity on all conceivable fronts. I applaud the various efforts driven toward this end.

Nevertheless, some human beings often take things too far. Predictably, their zealousness to cure social ills, as they define them, blur the lines and turn positives into negatives. If one closely follows typical media reports, it becomes readily apparent that words such as introspection, discipline, commitment and responsibility are most often attributed to the insensitive. This sends the wrong public message. It signals to the thoughtless, the undisciplined, the uncommitted and the irresponsible that nothing is their fault, and every bone-headed thought and deed in which they partake can be summarily dismissed due to a conveniently diagnosable condition. In short, nothing is anyone's fault—scapegoats abound. Heaven forbid that for the right reasons, not to shame or belittle, we dare to be honest and tell someone he's screwing up, didn't put in the effort or that he isn't qualified. Sensitivity and salving wounded feelings are all the rage today, at the expense of mental and physical development. Everyone gets a participation trophy because we are raising a nation of physical and mental weaklings; a nation of people who, for the most part, cannot deal with life.

Take the opioid crisis, for example. We constantly hear reports about the evil pharmaceutical companies placing profits over people, which I've already addressed, and irresponsible medical practitioners over-prescribing these terribly addictive and potentially deadly drugs. What we hardly, if ever, hear about are the thousands and thousands of jack-asses who are just looking to get high and subsequently become hooked on opioids. Suddenly, they are victims and have a disease. Victims and more victims. More often than not, one engages in foolish behavior first, then comes the so-called disease. For most, it's the same scenario when we're discussing alcohol and tobacco use. There is no cure for stupid.

When it comes to over-fat children, society is proceeding down the same mind-numbing path. It's interesting that whenever our children are threatened, as adults, we have a tendency to stand up and do something about it. This holds true unless the issue has to do with nutrition and fitness. Those of us who have been paying attention have heard repeatedly that this generation will probably be the first which does not have as long a life expectancy as their parents. The percentage of over-fat kids continues to soar along with the percentage of over-fat adults. I listen as newscasts announce the alarmingly rising incidences of children with type II diabetes, elevated cholesterol, elevated blood pressure and early markers for cardiovascular disease. Children needing to take medications that most adults, if they took care of themselves, wouldn't need, is a depressing testament to the kind of society we've become.

In addition to the dire physical consequences our children suffer due to being over-fat, the psychological effects can be just as impairing. Their social lives can be, and usually are, a living hell. The fat kid is the one who is most often bullied, mocked and picked last for teams by his schoolmates. Due to the stigma attached to over-fat children, it is assumed that these kids are lazy and sloppy. Many over-fat children suffer from depression and low self-esteem. Unless they are experiencing a severe case of denial, are clueless or simply don't give a damn, Americans know that the usual results of being over-fat are preventable disease, damage to one's psyche and premature death. These unpleasant yet predictable outcomes are the same for kids as they are for adults. I believe that most rational, honest people would generally agree that carrying around the excess fat that is prevalent among most people is undesirable.

The answer is not simply to teach the bullies not to make fun of the fat kid. I highly recommend lessons on civility, character and empathy be taught to all children. Yet, this strategy alone will not help the over-fat kid with his medical conditions, nor will it prevent the over-fat kid who is on the cusp of developing preventable diseases from acquiring these diseases.

So how do we prevent another generation of over-fat Americans from perpetuating another generation of over-fat Americans and so on and so on? The simple solution is that we must eat less and exercise more. Then why don't most of us utilize this simple solution? Because kids and adults need to first understand the causes encouraging their self-destructive behaviors prior to embarking on a wellness quest. Many explanations exist for their condition.

Most over-fat children spend more time sedentary than physically active. You can blame this on TV, video games, computers, the internet, smartphones and all manner of electronic devices connecting humanity to mindless social media. You can also blame parents tuned into current events, who watch a varied number of horrors unfold throughout the land on a daily basis. What responsible parent would not be afraid to allow their kids to run around outdoors, for fear of kidnappers, serial killers, terrorists, pedophiles and related cretins lurking behind every bush? When I was growing up in Newark, New Jersey, all the neighborhood kids played on the streets, in the parks and in playgrounds. Our moms had to repeatedly poke their heads out of windows, shouting for us to come home for dinner.

For the most part, only the weird kids stayed indoors all the time. Today, it seems that children don't know how to play, especially in suburbia. If suburban parents aren't living vicariously through their offspring and actively involved in their kid's playtime, setting up travel soccer, hockey, baseball and other athletic activities for their helpless youngsters, the kids are lost and don't know what to do. Parents act as chauffeurs, driving their kids everywhere. The children don't have to bike, let alone walk, anywhere.

This explanation works for the predicament of suburban kids, but what of urban kids? I still see plenty of them playing pickup games of various sports sans the overbearing eyes of their parents. So why are city kids fatter than those from years gone by? Perhaps it's due to the proliferation of fast food restaurants in urban neighborhoods. Also, many inner-city neighborhoods don't even have a halfway decent grocery store nearby, let alone a good market where wholesome, fresh produce can be purchased. Neighborhoods such as these are referred to by the media catchphrase "food deserts." Many of these communities should also be referred to as fast food oases. People need to eat to live. If relatively cheap, substandard foods are the only types conveniently available, the choices for these residents are obvious.

But remember, it's not just the poor and inner-city kids who are over-fat. Over-fatness cuts across all economic lines. Let's not get bogged down in a pointless discussion concerning which socioeconomic group has the greater percentage of over-fat kids. If we're being truthful with each other, the majority of all Americans are over-fat. Does anyone actually believe that wealthier people are not over-fat? Wealthy people are mostly educated and can model healthful behaviors for their kids. They usually don't. They have the means to join gyms and live in upscale communities where it's safe to exercise outdoors. They can easily afford to build home gyms if they so desire. The well-to-do can drive themselves and their children in their gas-guzzling status symbols on wheels to healthful food markets. They can afford any type of food they desire. What's their excuse for their over-fat kids, not to mention for their own corpulence?

Another frequently discussed reason for children becoming fatter today is that so many of them are products of households where both parents work. Everyone is busy, in a hurry, out of time and stressed. Parents arrive home late after a hectic day at work and then have to drive Junior to this practice or that function. Who has time to cook or eat together as a family? The adults, as well as their youngsters, grab whatever junk is most convenient, easily prepared and most pleasing to their taste buds. This serves as dinner, and off they go.

Non-availability of recreational facilities is another often-cited reason for the continuing expansion of our kids' girth. Yet, if you seek out and visit many playgrounds and athletic fields in various neighborhoods, you will, in fact, see facilities that are said to be nonexistent, but you will not see the kids utilizing them—it's the kids that don't exist.

Some blame the childhood obesity/overweight pandemic on genetics and their relationship with the environment. It is often stated that energy-frugal genes developed and proliferated in humans during ancient times when access to food was not guaranteed and unpredictable. According to this theory, these frugal genes helped our ancestors get through random famines. This fat gene remains with modern humans, but in the developed world, the environment has changed drastically from those long ago times. We now live in a world where vast amounts of food are available 24/7 all year long.

Even accepting the presence of this fat gene as a causative factor for certain people becoming over-fat is not an absolute and complete truth. It only serves as an excuse for a small number of people who have a propensity to become over-fat. At best, it's a partial explanation and a minor one at that. I contend that for the energy-frugal gene to gain a foothold and do its damage, it most often requires a welcoming bodily environment to manifest. Consuming substandard food, lack of exercise and other unhealthful behaviors provides such an environment.

The reasons provided for why kids and adults alike continue to become over-fat proliferate almost as rapidly as the fat pounds accumulate on these same people. I recall talk of a "fat virus" over 10 years ago. However, even the individuals who were espousing this hypothesis maintained that while it was a convenient excuse for gaining unwanted weight, it was a poor and inadequate explanation for the majority of America's skyrocketing over-fat problem.

256

Poverty is another oft-cited reason for childhood obesity/overweight. I've lost track of the number of articles I've read and news reports I've heard asserting that impoverishment is at the root cause of this problem. These types of reports usually focus on the disparate conditions and environments dividing the well-to-do and the poor black, brown and rural white kids. A typical report is replete with cumbersome statistics comparatively pinpointing salaries, percentages of children afflicted and geographic locations.

Childhood obesity/overweight is said to be a complicated dilemma induced by numerous affairs. I generally agree that the reasons for this predicament are multifaceted. Poverty, geography and limited education all enable our children to continue to pack on unhealthful weight. Regardless of this fact, Americans allow themselves to get bogged down in the numbers and statistics game promoted by experts, the authorities and the media, but what's the point?

With the preponderance of helpful information that can be easily accessed and the sheer common sense nature of what, at minimum, healthful living entails, why are educated people over-fat? Why are wealthy people burdened with unhealthful weight gain? Why are people who live in nice suburban neighborhoods eating themselves into a coma? Why do fun, frivolity and general good times almost always revolve around "I know I shouldn't" and "this is so sinful" type foods, all washed down with alcohol? Why do adults not see or perhaps simply refuse to accept the fact of the miserable example they set for their children?

Yes, statistics depict children as well as adults of certain races and ethnic groups to be at higher risk for unwanted weight gain than others. What are we to do, engage in an endless political and uninspired war of statistics, numbers, charts and graphs and solve nothing, as per usual? Let's get real here, America; there are plenty of unhealthy fat people in just about every segment of society we've deemed necessary to separate from the greater whole. Open your eyes, almost everyone is unhealthfully fat!

It's all been said and done to the point where I'd like all the experts, all the politicians and everyone else who is supposedly "waging war" on childhood obesity/overweight and overweight in general to please stop talking. They aren't helping, continue to fail with aplomb, yet they prattle on. They should spare us the nonsense. Americans aren't responsible enough to keep their pets from getting fat, and we should be astonished that their children are permitted to inflate like dirigibles? So what, if a particularly designated group, categorized, codified and otherwise indexed by the U.S. Census Bureau or other lumbering governmental bureaucracy has a higher or lower percentage of unhealthy fat kids? They all need help. Unfortunately, the stats are what the media sink their teeth into, distracting the population from the overall nature of the problem, while providing the people with useless talking points leading to the usually perpetuated false narratives.

As it happens, most of the people pointing fingers at obese and overweight children while clamoring for solutions are themselves over-fat. But of course, they're not obese, only socially acceptable fat. They, too, should be quiet because they have no credibility. They need to look into a mirror if they dare. It seems to me that a disproportionate number of adults and organizations who purport to wage war on childhood obesity in America and the over-fat epidemic in general refuse to acknowledge that responsibility and choices play the major role in gaining unhealthful, excess weight. While the various reasons I mentioned in the continuing supersizing of America play a part, their role is less significant than those running the show would have the population believe. This makes the people feel better about themselves because there is always someone or something else to blame for their foolishness. The people require honest information, not coddling, not more excuses.

Because most of the population has at least a rudimentary idea of what constitutes healthful behavior, lecturing them, at this point, on the dangers of being over-fat and unfit is nothing short of a ridiculous public service announcement. It's no better than reminding those woebegone souls to place the fork into their mouth rather than into an eye when eating because of the extreme possibility of damaging their vision by sticking the fork into an eye. Too much obvious information and no one is listening. Discovering that one, two or eleven more really horrific things will most likely happen to us and to our children, who are on the road to becoming us, as a result of over-fat, will not make one bit of difference. What more do we need to know? It can't get much worse than allowing yourself and your children to become overweight and then coming to grips with the idea that you dropping dead of a heart attack at age 40 is a very real possibility. That you can develop certain cancers and watch your body consume itself, have an appendage lopped off due to complications from diabetes or have a blood vessel explode in your head are, indeed, grim possibilities. If these potential scenarios don't encourage relatively reasonable adults to change their self-destructive habits, fearing for themselves, as well as for the dismal future they've engineered for their children, nothing will.

When we're not busy playing the victim and making excuses for our moronic behaviors, the real reasons for childhood obesity and mostly everyone's overweight, in general, filters through into our collective consciousness. They have been enumerated repeatedly for decades now. As a country, we are as familiar with these reasons as we are with the consequences of over-fat. For those who are not, it's because they've not been paying attention, don't care, are delusional or are in absolute denial.

In review, the reasons for childhood obesity/overweight that are being spoon-fed to the public look something like this:

1. We live in a high-tech world in which kids sit too long watching TV, playing video games and are glued to smartphones and other devices engaging in mindless social media. They're in their homes instead of burning calories and building muscle while running about outdoors. I know plenty of techno-geek kids who are not over-fat.

2. Kids who live in the suburbs don't like to walk anywhere anymore because their parents drive them everywhere. I know many kids who are driven to their various activities who are not over-fat.

3. City kids are overweight because there are too many fast-food restaurants around and not enough decent grocery stores. The city kids are simultaneously not fat because they are outside playing numerous types of pickup games in playgrounds, parks and on the streets. But they are also fat because there are not enough recreational facilities to fill their needs.

4. Rural kids are overweight because, umm...let's see, they have plenty of outdoor space, they can play outside because crime is so much lower than in cities, and there are no conveniently accessible fast-food restaurants in their areas. Oh yeah, but they also spend the same inordinate amount of time engaged with their social media devices in the same brain-shriveling activities as their counterparts in cities.

5. Kids are fat because they come from poor homes. My father was fat as a kid; a child of poor immigrants. He had three siblings and none of them were fat. So, my father was fat because he was poor, and his brothers and sister were thin because they were poor.

6. Some kids are over-fat because they are members of a minority race or ethnicity. Even if some statistics bear out that a higher percentage of these children are over-fat, so what? Fat is fat. The reality is that fat kids inhabit every group. Predictably, playing the race or ethnic card will not help these struggling youngsters. Let's look at this situation as having two groups—

healthy, fit kids and sickly, unfit kids. Overfat hurts all kids. No matter their race or ethnicity, they all suffer equally.

7. The "both parents work" theory is another allegation for why kids become fat. When I was a little kid, only my father worked. My mother was a stay-at-home mom. I have two sisters; all three of us were fat. As we three siblings became older children, my mom went back to work. We became a "both parents work" household. My sisters and I, despite both parents working, became un-fat.

8. Genetics make kids fat. While it may be accurate that some children have a genetic predisposition for becoming over-fat, this makes little difference, if they are active and properly nourished. At any rate, only an extremely small percentage of any group is over-fat due to genetic predisposition. Do you really believe that practically 75% of the country has become over-fat as the result of a DNA problem? It may make you more comfortable to embrace this reasoning, but that will not make it so. Most, not all, but most people become over-fat as a result of poor nutritional choices and a lack of meaningful exercise. In the case of those ill-fated children, lack of training, lack of education and appalling adult role models are the primary culprits causing their excess fat.

9. A virus makes kids fat. While this may be possible, the kids who become fat due to a virus are undoubtedly infinitesimal in number.

After having read the reasons for our nation's childhood/overweight tsunami, are you as confused as I am? How can you not be? Some of the aforementioned reasons for childhood obesity/over-fat are not without a small degree of merit. Despite this, it's unfortunate that these hackneyed excuses and similar ones are presented to the masses as gospel. They provide an easy, guiltless way out and, thus, avoid placing the responsibility where it belongs—on parents and on an educational system that talks a good game but is, in reality, indifferent about the nutritional needs and fitness of our youth. The message being delivered over and over is that it's not your fault because you are simply a victim.

When a society is replete with not only parents and educators but saturated with an overwhelmingly popular attitude about a subject, an attitude which is in clear evidence simply by observing the general condition of its population, it becomes extremely difficult to change the standard belief system. Societal opportunists are always astute as to which way the wind is blowing and give the majority what it wants. Kids don't have much of a chance in this scenario.

Unless they've been living under a rock somewhere for the last 50 years, most Americans, although they have a difficult time accepting it, are well aware of the perils of being unfit and over-fat. This is because the very same system that encourages us to eat junk food, drink alcohol and other junk beverages, and to engage in all manner of potentially self-harming behaviors simultaneously warns us against the practice of these behaviors. However, the system warns us in the most muted way possible, perhaps not wanting the people to turn away from it. The system wants to have it both ways, ensuring that all bases are covered. As a result, it can claim that it was providing good information even if things go wrong. A good example is cigarette companies showing us how cool it is to smoke while at the same time placing health warnings about smoking cigarettes on the packaging.

Researchers will continue to search for other culprits causing childhood, as well as adult, over-fat. Many of the over-fat and unfit grownups will continue to unearth their own justifications for their plight. Very little, if any, of this madness will help the children. I'll say it again: the vast majority of kids are fat and unfit not due to a virus, genetics or any other lame excuse, but because they were never trained in the importance of proper nutrition and meaningful exercise. How could they have possibly been trained? The adults, whose care these children depend upon, are as irresponsible as the children themselves. The children have a legitimate excuse—they're children. The adults, not so much.

It's also important to mention that many youngsters who are not carrying around unwanted body fat also eat substandard food, consume sugary drinks and may be physically inactive. This has its own set of problems which most people can't begin to wrap their silly heads around. Looking fine on the outside doesn't automatically mean that one's insides are not being destroyed as a consequence of poor behaviors. We are all so involved in the fat discussion that we fail to recognize that this is only one aspect of a much larger human problem—we engage in a preponderance of behaviors that are potentially and outright harmful to our well-being while giving the health consequences nary a thought. It can be argued that the childhood obesity/overweight problem in this country is complex. I would disagree. While there are plenty of bad actors and enablers who share in the blame of perpetuating a fat, unfit America, I contend that if we keep addressing the multifacetedness of the problem, we will not be able to get out of our own way in order to solve it. We've overcomplicated an elementary societal problem, i.e., most people don't take care of their health. It's a simple fix which requires a commitment we are unwilling to muster.

Average people regularly allow themselves to be manipulated. However, if you desire to improve your health and the health of your children and to set a baseline of good health in preparation for what may come, you need to take responsibility for your actions. At some point, no matter your description or governmental characterization, you need to stop lying to yourself. Only then will you stop playing the victim in this long, sad story.

Society is controlled by adults, not children. The adults are the real cause of childhood obesity/overweight. This is due to the society they created for the kids. With some assistance and a bit of luck, a few youngsters manage to navigate the self-destructive, anti-nutrition and anti-health advocacies promoted by the innumerable adult-run mechanisms in society. These kids don't fall prey to the prodigious forces compelling them to make self-harming choices. This isn't because it's easy, but because of the training and luck I just mentioned and their strength of will. Weaker-minded kids, those easily led, are prime candidates for exploitation due to their lack of will and self-confidence. Shameless, remorseless adults and the anti-health apparatus they control will continue to bombard our children with their endless stream of lies, wishy-washy solutions, encouragements and calculating tactics.

Sugary junk cereals, vaping, soda, tobacco, alcohol, tanning beds, fast food, junk food and countless other products, along with their associated consumption or use, have been, for far too long, romanticized and portrayed in a positive and fun-filled light. We experience this insanity every day. To reframe what I stated earlier, childhood/obesity is much more than just that. Our kids don't know how to make wise health decisions. This goes far beyond nutritional choices alone because the adults have failed them in spectacular fashion. The adults have their own individual agendas—health, in general, is an afterthought.

These same adults, those who set the groundwork for childhood over-fat, as well as most of the other problems afflicting our youth, are the quickest to jump on the bandwagon to decry the situation and pontificate about the pain and suffering caused by childhood obesity. It makes them appear concerned. The childhood obesity pandemic is a hot topic and never too far removed from the headlines. It keeps these supposedly concerned individuals relevant. The problem gets worse and worse as they talk on.

Every now and then we hear about how some locally isolated movements in various sectors of American society, including some schools and communities, have succeeded in making a variety of nutritional and fitness improvements for kids. I applaud and encourage all such efforts.

Nevertheless, they are like a voice in the wilderness. Many of these endeavors meet with great resistance from the supporters of the status quo. The reality is that other than a few disconnected skirmishes being fought in far-flung outposts of the country, the actual war against childhood obesity has yet to begin.

The response to this scourge upon our youth has been insipid and fraught with political correctness and social niceties. It has not been nearly enough. Both official and unofficial reactions are moving at the pace of a tortoise, if at all, while the number of over-fat kids bounds ahead at the speed of the proverbial hare.

I'll go back to education. Education at school, at home, on the airwaves, in print and on social media to inspire a new paradigm is what is desperately needed. We don't need more "love yourself no matter what" drivel. If humans don't seek enlightenment in thought and deed, in short, improvement, what's the point to just be, even at the expense of our health and that of our children? Yes, self-love is the keystone to a life of contentment, but not the way it is popularly being interpreted and presented. We should love ourselves enough to care about our health and well-being—controlling what we can. Allowing ourselves and our children to become over-fat, thus opening the door to diseases that are easily preventable, has nothing to do with loving oneself and everything to do with indulging dangerous wants. The current presentation and promotion of loving oneself is wrapped in a feel-good shroud. It's a copout and ignores the catastrophic consequences of excess body fat wrought by nutritionally poor food choices. To be clear, I'm strictly speaking about things one can control.

Most adults are set in their ways. The real hope lies with our children. This hope will only be realized if enough adults are willing to come to grips with this problem and display true leadership, something which has been in dreadfully short supply. If the authorities were serious about this issue, they would cease their rhetoric and take dramatic and decisive action. We need fresh, radical solutions. The health of our children deserves nothing less because, in most cases, over-fat causes diseases and early death. Our schools, grades K through 12, need to implement mandatory daily nutrition and fitness education classes which are on par with those subjects traditionally perceived to be more important (they're not): math, science, and English.

Every manner of junk food and junk drink needs to be eliminated from school grounds, including the cafeteria, hallway vending machines and class parties. Schools need to seek other sources of funding for resurfacing their athletic fields or sending the band to a competition out of state. Schools prostituting themselves and, as a result, placing our children at risk by signing contracts allowing purveyors of disease-promoting drinks and snacks to place their vending machines in school hallways must end. All prospective teachers, not only those seeking certification in nutrition, fitness and wellness education, need to be taught about the great importance of nutrition and exercise. This would be an easy sell if the foundation had already been laid when they were youngsters in primary and secondary schools.

Teachers, such as these would be formidable educators. It's very easy to intertwine nutritional lessons when teaching the standard subjects. Think of the critical thought required, the classroom discussions and the wonderful writing assignments that would actively engage the students. Utilizing English, social studies, math and other disciplines to demonstrate to kids how they are preyed upon by unscrupulous, money-hungry corporations would go a long way toward preventing another generation of sick kids.

These ideas, and similar ones, would constitute a real start to seriously addressing the childhood obesity/overweight pandemic. An initiative such as what I've described would demonstrate to the public the seriousness of the problem. This guidance would also cause exponentially positive societal results. Other ideas, efforts and programs would flow from this foundation. Intellectually, most of what we learn happens in school. The parents of the children we seek to educate were also educated in schools. Parents and kids influence one another. Schools need to establish themselves as the bedrock of proper nutrition, exercise and overall wellness education. They need to push back strongly against the noise pollution generated by the media, advertisers and disingenuous food producers. We need this initial flow of change to become a title wave of solutions.

Our governmental authorities and bureaucrats need to decide whether or not they are willing to sacrifice a bit of economic growth. This translates to giant corporations being satisfied with individually raking in, for example, "only" $20 billion in profits this year, as opposed to the $30 billion in profits they made last year. Politicians and policymakers must be willing to sacrifice their popularity for the well-being of our kids. Do these politicos have the gumption to anger those corporations whose influence and money helped get them elected and kept them in office by admitting that these same corporations are contributing to the deterioration of the health of our kids? In order to help future generations, something we so often hear about, our belief system regarding nutrition, fitness and healthful behaviors in general needs a revisionist approach. The traditional ways are simply not getting it done.

The childhood obesity problem and obesity in general do not seem to be improving. Each time I step out into public, it appears to be worsening. This has been going on for generations because we've allowed it. Think about that for a minute. I realize that the wheels of government turn slowly and that our leaders need to be prudent so as not to make rash decisions. However, it's been decades, and we've yet to make significant and meaningful strides which would enable us to boast about our victory concerning this outrageous problem.

Our children are suffering from maladies not normally seen until they throw in the towel just after middle age and become fat, sick, old people. Now we have fat, sick, old-like people who are young. This is unacceptable in a modern, civilized, intelligent society and should make the citizenry mad as hell. Each year, the percentage of over-fat kids shows every sign of increasing. However, I sometimes hear reports about how this percentage has stabilized. I don't believe these reports because I have eyes. Further, stabilization should be considered a good thing? Stabilized at what, 20%, 30%, 40%, depending on which report we choose to accept and who performed the study? This won't bring much comfort to those residing in the stabilized group.

Every year, the government wrings its hands, expresses concern, initiates another study and revises its dietary guidelines. Enough! We, the people, need to take matters into our own hands and act in our own best self-interest and in the interest of our children. It is imperative that we apply pressure for governmental reforms and through personal actions and inactions, such as refusing to line the pockets of manufacturers by not purchasing their disease-promoting products. Except for those very few isolated outposts of grass-roots sanity I mentioned a few paragraphs ago, in this vast wasteland of nutritional ignorance and apathy, very little has been accomplished in the battle of our nation's bulge. What small victories have been won were hard-fought against established governmental institutions in league with entrenched behaviors, further interwoven into the very fabric of our culture. To the enlightened few, I urge you to carry on. But more of us need to do more because our kids soon run out of time. The powers that be are not dependable. Their policies are no more than a Band-Aid on a critical wound that requires life-saving, emergency surgery. In other words, their efforts fall grievously short and bring about very little that is of consequence. The responsibility for eradicating childhood obesity/over-fat ultimately rests on the shoulders of we, the common citizens.

56

In Review

We are a country that professes the importance of education. Yet, when the topic turns to nutrition, fitness and health, we wallow in our own ignorance. We are self-made victims of every weight-loss gimmick that comes down the pike, only to be disappointed by their inevitable inability to solve our problem. Nonetheless, this disappointment does little to deter us from our nonsensical stubbornness in attempting the next miracle weight-loss or get-fit product that the never-ending number of hucksters are eagerly willing to provide to the pathetic and desperately out-of-shape. We never get it.

This situation is bad enough for adults to experience, but at least adults have the opportunity to choose. What choice does a young child or a baby have? Straight from the womb, we immediately begin a child's indoctrination into the prevailing, sick societal system that influenced the majority of us, producing a nation of fat, medicated, educated fools. As we go bumbling and stumbling about, whining that we can't lose those extra pounds, making one excuse after another, compounded by repeated silly choices, we continue the very same dumb behaviors. This is the example we set for our children—most of whom, under current conditions, don't have a chance in hell of growing up to become anything other than over-fat, over-medicated grownups, just like mom and dad.

You might say that at least the institutions that are responsible for teaching our kids will pick up the slack where ignorant parents left off, right? If you believe this, you are so very wrong. As I touched on earlier, it should be that way, but it's not. Our schools, for the most part, are fairly adept at teaching traditional subjects, including reading, math, science and many other important and interesting subjects, which were not available when I was in school. However, what good is all this knowledge if your use of it is cut short because of debilitating illness or premature death? If you weren't taught how healthful habits can significantly prolong a healthful life, traditional education seems hollow.

I stand by the proclamation that nothing is more important than health. Knowledge concerning a particular subject makes no difference, nor do a multitude of earned degrees from prestigious universities. I'm not impressed by exorbitant salaries or by job descriptions. The ability to sit all day long and pontificate with pinpoint knowledge about affairs of state, international relations, economics, nuclear physics, biochemistry, religion, politics, sports or the arts does not move me. Being well versed in all the fields I've just listed, although unlikely, possessing a PhD from Princeton and having achieved billionaire status to boot, in my eyes, is worthless if the individual is an over-fat, unfit tragedy waiting to happen. Health trumps all.

We live in a mostly artificial world that is becoming increasingly more artificial. The masses seek to further escape, as a result of technology, into more deeply artificial worlds. These worlds are built by mostly physically weak, albeit academically intelligent people, who require titles, institutions, status and money to keep them insulated in a state of manufactured power and in a position of control. But in the end, the only real power, the only thing we possess that is really worth anything, is our healthy selves.

Humans, with our oversized hubrises, refuse to acknowledge what fragile creatures we are. We can be killed or can suddenly and unexpectedly die so easily. We can cease to exist in a flash by forces beyond our control. Yet, we insist on increasing the odds, favoring our early termination by our idiotic behaviors. So often, we hear about the sanctity of life, but the reality seems to be that those words only apply when mass murderers or oppressive regimes are involved in the killing. These sorts of atrocities garner headlines, whereas people slowly killing themselves year after year, by the hundreds of thousands, as a result of bodily deterioration from terrible food choices, a lack of significant exercise and other questionable behaviors elicits a mostly apathetic response.

We may be individually special to our loved ones, but overall, how special can humans be if, in the end, we are reduced to nothing more than stinking, rotting meat? In the light of harsh reality, no one but a handful of people really give a damn about each of us. More so, the reason why we, on an individual basis, should give a damn about ourselves by committing to vigorously protecting our health. If you're lucky, you are special to a few people who love you. Ultimately, you should be special to yourself because you're all you have.

Americans, and all people living in similar societies, must awaken and develop survival instincts, enabling them to cast aside the chains keeping them tethered to the values of cultures guilty of inundating them with propaganda every day. The load of these unseen chains is felt by those gullible enough to acquiesce to the ideas, euphemisms and fabrications of political and corporate powers. The benevolence of these political and corporate monoliths goes only as far as it serves their own needs. If their needs do little to serve you and instead foster and/or sustain a sick culture, so be it. This culture is one where politicians and corporate honchos reign supreme,

267

where we have allowed it to manipulate us into all manner of self-destructive behaviors as we stand around, feeble, in the face of societal coercions. We cheer the next trendy catchphrase and eloquent speech. We embrace them as if these words will make a difference to our pitiful condition. We will dance in the streets, living it up, so to speak, partying and observing our own demise. By the time we realize what we've empowered the colossus to do to us and what we've done to ourselves, it will be too late.

We are constantly conditioned by society to think and behave in particular ways that, on the surface, appear to benefit all. The power and money-grabbing elite have always attempted to benefit themselves through, in one way or another, control of the common citizens, including a desire to predict our behavior. For the most part, they have succeeded. We have aided and abetted our self-serving overlords by joining with them and partaking in their ideas and products. We have permitted them into duping us into becoming simple tools to advance their agendas. We have lost all sense of critical thought and introspection. We are miserable and confounded, physical wrecks, as are many of those very same individuals who benefit from our stupid decisions. We have run away from what we are. Yes, we are human beings, but we are animals. Denying what we are does not make us something else. We are flesh and blood, like other animals.

The fact that we are animals can be seen in our genetic code. The continuation of all living creatures, including man, hinges on survival of the fittest. We stand a much better chance of remaining fit and healthy through proper nutrition and exercise—not by gorging on inferior, sickness-inducing products and lying about like fat slugs, toying with our electronic devices.

If we continue to be sheep and act upon the designs of the puppet masters who have happily shepherded us into our present corral of unfitness, we will certainly face a life, no doubt a shortened one, of sickness, pain, impediments and self-imposed torment. Rational beings don't consider this to be what living is about, and it's certainly not what they want for their children. To survive and thrive, we must remain true to our animal nature—not succumb to deceitful temptation.

When governments deem an issue important enough, they enact legislation and policy to address it. At the very least, they offer public service announcements to keep the public informed. Governments, more so than ordinary citizens, can do just about what they want to, even when restricted by laws. They have much bigger and better toolboxes containing everything from hammers to finely honed blades which can be wielded, not only by their members, but by governmental lawyers, with equal proficiency. Governments add, repeal, modify and otherwise mold policies to suit their needs. On the rare occasion when bipartisanism comes about, action is taken relatively quickly. When there is disagreement among political factions in government and in the population, as is usually the case, the wheels of government get bogged down in a mire of red tape, overlapping policies, bureaucratic double-speak, conflicting legislation and, at times, a wild west of no regulations at all. Many times, these governmental actions or inactions, as the case may be, do little to resolve the concern and have little effect on your well-being and survival. This is especially and clearly evident when nutrition and fitness are the topics.

We must stop waiting for help and help ourselves. The minority of people who actually comprehend the benefits of a healthful way of life and practice it need to stand up and apply pressure on elected officials, school boards and policymakers. Still, we need not idly wait for the authorities to act. While we're applying pressure via phone calls, letters, editorials, social media, peaceful protests and other assorted grass-roots movements, not acting also sends a powerful message. What I'm referring to is the non-act of buying garbage foods and beverages. Could you imagine the message that would be sent to the elites if the common people worked together for their mutual benefit, chose one lousy product, and simply refused to ever buy it again? That would be a world-changing movement on the right side of history. The time for moving slowly was yesterday. Action is what's needed—now.

More than a few public school teachers with whom I am acquainted have long complained about a lack of fundamental teaching in their respective schools due to ongoing and seemingly endless preparations for standardized testing, a testing culture which shifted into a much higher gear about 25 years ago. They have stated they have little time for anything else other than test prep, testing, and gathering and chronicling the resultant data. It's not unusual for many a teacher to be hunched over a home computer well after midnight, tediously logging in and reporting that data on various bureaucratic forms, only to have to rise in a few hours, go to work and continue the madness.

With shit invariably traveling downhill, members of local boards of education quake in fear of losing their positions. They are compelled to pressure school administrators, who also live in fear of losing their jobs, who in turn push teachers who fear losing their jobs if the standardized testing and required documents are not completed, as per federally mandated deadlines and edicts. It's common knowledge in the field of education that, in many cases, the results of standardized tests have a significant effect on school funding. The ones who benefit most from these tests are the school testing corporations, not the students. It is an industry that has grown into a giant since its humble beginnings in the 1950s. In America, big business and making money supersede education—this is what's prioritized. Finding a way to add real nutrition and fitness courses to school curricula does not take precedence.

As you can see, when it wants to, governments can amend rules in the middle of the game. Americans who care about a healthy population need to force their government's hand by applying pressure on the numerous fronts that impact our health. We can begin by demanding nutrition and fitness education in our nation's schools. Physical and health education have been downsized, if not completely eliminated, for all practical purposes in most of our public schools. What I'm suggesting is not a continuation or return to what passed for physical education when I was in school. Most of the teachers I remember were lazy, over-fat physical specimens who would just throw out the balls, allowing the athletic kids to dominate the choosing of teams, as well as the actual games.

The talented kids beat the crap out of the less talented fat kids, who were reluctantly picked for teams and always last. It's no wonder the less athletic kids hated gym class. Physical education was nothing more than a forum for the athletically gifted to further showcase their talents and for the athletically challenged to get embarrassed. It was hard enough to be a kid as it was, without the anticipatory terrors plaguing the over-fat, sports-challenged in preparation for the ignominious situation in which they would soon find themselves. There was not a great deal of physical education going on back then. These instructors were not, and never would be, the type of people who kids looked to as role models. What little preaching they were doing, they were clearly not practicing. Students were less than inspired to improve their fitness because the hypocrisy was blatant.

Health education was no better. I had a health teacher in high school who taught, loosely speaking, the class with an unlit cigar clenched between his teeth. If you plan on a career as a physical education or health teacher, you need to be a true believer in these disciplines. Posers, or worse yet, detractors, don't steer the students in the right direction. Far too many so-called physical education and health teachers, past and present, were and continue to exist, as does the majority of the rest of society, in a state of over-fat and unfitness. People such as these shouldn't be certified in this type of subject matter. They should teach subjects where the educator's physical appearance and health has no direct correlation to the subject matter being taught.

As I've mentioned throughout, people are constantly repeating the "everything in moderation" mantra, particularly when discussing eating and exercise. We don't teach math, history, spelling, language or the sciences in moderation. Why is it that when it comes to our knowledge of nutrition and fitness, the word moderation enters into the vernacular? Nutrition, fitness and overall wellness practices, the most important subjects we can learn because they have a direct impact on life and death, are not courses to be taught in moderation by disinterested parties. That's like being enrolled in a survival course taught by someone whose behaviors ensure that he will not survive. This subject matter needs to be presented honestly and not necessarily gently by people who live by their principles and convictions if it is expected to have any real impact on the student body.

I'm sure some will argue that moderation is key to nutrition and fitness education because there are so many varying opinions regarding what actually constitutes proper food and exercise. To these individuals, I would submit that plenty of divergent opinions are routinely floated concerning how particular historical events "really" unfolded. Scientific studies may have numerous interpretations, various dialects exist of their mother language, and opinions abound dealing with who, what or if God really is. The disparities of opinion never cause someone to state that these interests need to be taught in moderation.

The body and mind are both components of a single unit: you. They both require nurturing and education in order to evolve into something higher, better and more significant. Who was it that decided nurturing and educating the mind and allowing the body to fall by the wayside was a good idea? If the body gets sick and dies, the mind dies as well. In a self-abused, sick and unfit body, traditional academics serve only as partial learning. Traditional academics are not the most important kind of knowledge. You can acquire all the traditional book learning you desire, but if you are over-fat and unfit, that knowledge will not help you avoid early disease and death. You're rolling the dice and betting with your life.

If I were in charge (and I'm certain some of you are breathing a sigh of relief that I'm not), I would propose a mandatory, age-appropriate nutrition, fitness and overarching health education curriculum in all schools, beginning in preschool and lasting through high school. It would include courses that teach the purpose of eating, how to eat properly, what not to eat, effects of poor dietary choices, nutrition and disease prevention, pesticides on produce, food processing, forums on the various diets that receive so much hype, how food is marketed—especially to kids in that they represent the prime targets of manipulative advertising practices, how politics play a role in the

271

food we eat by way of farm subsidies and many other potential topics. Course materials would also include honest and straightforward discussions regarding smoking and tobacco products, vaping, caffeine, recreational drugs, and the most significant recreational drug of all, alcohol. In addition, classes would instruct the students on proper exercise protocols, including how to devise comprehensive workout routines, explanations of different types of exercise modalities and their purposes. The classes would also include basic physiology and anatomy.

Further, every student would participate in a physical education class at the beginning of the school day. I'm not talking about the pointless running around we did. What I'm referring to is one hour of working out five days per week, every week. Children need to be taught that working out each day is as important as brushing their teeth. It must be a routine part of life. Kids need to be able to defend their health by preparing mentally and physically for the onslaught of those who mislead them.

My schools would stop rewarding students with junk food for a job well done. These supposed rewards, so prevalent today, in the form of sugary cookies, cheesy pizza parties, soda and artery-clogging, fat-inducing cupcakes, set the stage for the development of habits that will have long-lasting, detrimental health effects on the children as they mature. Today's children have been conditioned by people they trust to believe that there is nothing wrong with these types of foods. This makes it extremely difficult for the kids to improve their future health. They accept this garbage as normal food. Sadly, in a sense, it is to them.

We talk a good game about how we care about the health and safety of our children. Yet, we allow machines in our schools that dispense soda, juice drinks, sports drinks and other assorted junk drinks, in addition to a wide variety of junk foods. Schools are where children go to acquire knowledge. When we permit junk drinks and junk foods in schools, we are sending mixed messages to young, developing minds. Hypocrisy is the lesson being taught here. My proposal would eliminate all of these vending machines from school property. The appropriate authorities need to be forced by intelligent, concerned parents to do so. I don't care how many millions of dollars a particular beverage company may offer a school for exclusive pouring rights. Accepting this money is morally and ethically wrong.

I'm well aware that when school budgets fall short, they use this money to pay for everything from technological equipment for computer labs to synthetic turf for athletic fields. Schools that follow this practice whore themselves by allowing these purveyors of pestilence to place their poisons on school property in exchange for a big payday. Authorizing these companies to advertise on school grounds or permitting them to sponsor school events is not much better. These practices may serve as short-term fixes for financial problems but at the expense of long-term, healthful outcomes for the kids. Some argue the elimination of exclusive pouring rights and other school vending machine contracts will cause local property taxes to increase to pay for school improvements. This just goes to show how broken the system is. Tough decisions are required to repair it, but we must begin somewhere. Schools will just have to make do without the extras until a fair and reasonable method of funding is devised. It is absolutely unreasonable to place the health of our children at risk to achieve this end.

Most food being served in schools is putrid, be it cafeteria food or the low-cost and free meals being provided to students. It is dominated by unhealthful, sugary, salty, fat-laden and chemically infused dreck, masquerading and touted as healthful fare. Improvements are being made in some parts of the country, but they remain few and far between. The government would have the population believe that school food is improving dramatically by feeding one success story to the media, who then blare out the wonderful headlines. The sad truth is that improvements in school food are but isolated occurrences.

The fact that kids are permitted to choose between healthful food and unhealthful food, especially in the cafeteria, is preposterous. Sure, let them choose, but ensure that all the offerings are of the healthful variety. Some say that the children don't like this. Tough, they're not in charge. They will thank you later in life. School nutritionists and dietitians know in their hearts and by way of their education what constitutes healthful and what doesn't, so let's stop playing games. I've already mentioned junk drinks. We can add flavored milk, chocolate and strawberry, for example, to the junk drink list. These wholesome-sounding beverages contain as much, if not more, sugar than some sodas. If it were up to me, I'd do away with all animal milk. But the dairy industry and dairy lobby in America is a story unto itself. Suffice to say, I'm not a fan.

One of the numerous problems with school food is that the federal government is involved. This would be fine if the federal government had a reputation for efficiency, transparency and for making sound decisions based on the welfare of the people instead of caving into politics and business. Government officials boast about all the good they are doing, but in reality, they're supporting something very bad by permitting unhealthful food in schools. Official websites concerning school food are peppered with bureaucratic jargon and legalese and are tedious to read.

They contain very little information describing what the best foods are. It's all very official and important sounding and is intended to depict the government as the great savior, stepping in to rescue the children from going hungry. Their solution is to fill the bellies of kids with bad food.

The federal government guidelines for school meal programs require schools to serve the bad food they, in fact, serve. Otherwise, federal funding for the schools' meal programs will be affected. So of course, from a local school board point of view, everyone concerned acquiesces to the mandates of the federal government. This is one of the main reasons why it is so difficult to "exorcise" bad food from schools and replace it with proper food. This will only occur when a large portion of the population protests loudly and consistently enough, causing politicians to fear for their jobs.

A hot dog, French fries, sugary fruit cup and strawberry-flavored cow milk may satisfy the low bar nutritional standards written up by some expert bureaucrat, but that sure as hell doesn't make this rubbish healthful. Throw in the candy-like, mainstream cereals and pastries that are a routine part of school breakfasts, and the absurdity of school food comes further into focus. There is no rational argument against this point. The only thing worse than what typically passes for healthful school food is you, the parent, believing that it's healthful and allowing your child to consume it. Educate yourself, then protest vociferously, as if your kid's life depends on it—because it does.

There are always going to be those children, just like adults, who don't like particular foods and have an aversion to physical activity. We place too much emphasis on what kids like or may not like and not enough emphasis on what's best for them in the long run. Most of us didn't like algebra, but it was still required. We can't please everyone, so we shouldn't try to. What we need to do is what's right. Children need to be taught about the benefits of delayed gratification. They must learn when to use and why they use that part of their brain that thinks slowly and critically, as during academic and intellectual discussions, for example. On the other hand, kids need to be taught to keep their instant reward-seeking, quick-thinking, primitive brains in check unless it needs to be engaged, as in times of danger. Because younger children usually want to please their teachers, they are more malleable and, therefore, more inclined to accept and adopt positive health habits. As such, it's critical to begin training them in these positive health habits at the onset of their school enrollment. If this training begins in preschool and continues through grades K-12, it becomes the new normal, as do the positive health outcomes it fosters. Nutritional recalcitrance, in later years, will be dramatically diminished and marginalized, as is slowly but steadily happening with cigarette smokers.

It's obvious that adults are skilled at teaching children how to do things the wrong way, as evidenced by the losing war being waged on childhood over-fat. The type of nutrition and fitness education our children have received to this point has been spiritless. It has been provided by ignorant parents, an impotent and disinterested school system, a money-driven media, and further perpetuated by a bunch of self-serving, agenda-fueled politicians and policymakers. If this kind of so-called education is not immediately stopped, our kids will only continue to learn how to harm themselves. As a result of their self-injurious conditioning, they will, in turn, pass their flawed knowledge and habits of self-torment to their offspring, just as it was passed on to them. This is a surefire way of ensuring that the suffering will continue.

At what point do we stop the lunacy? What is the price we must pay? How many more American kids must be encouraged to begin killing themselves or to be ushered into adulthood as sick adults who will assuredly require multiple medications and, just as assuredly, die prematurely? How much more nonsense will we tolerate? How much more anguish can we sustain until a sober mass of people rise up and protest in disgust? Has the obesity/over-fat plague in our country not made itself evident enough? Don't the legions of fat kids with adult-like health issues provide ample proof of the tragic scope of overindulgence inundating our land?

How much more corroboration do Americans require before the realization sets in that their attitudes about nutrition and fitness are killing their children, as well as themselves? What more verification is necessary? Do we need to suffer more strokes, diabetes, heart disease, cancer, hypertension, discouragement and self-contradictory behavior to illuminate the miserable distinction between the senseless exhortations of a sick culture and what is actually beneficial for the population, including our kids? As the iconic and brilliant Crosby, Stills, Nash & Young sang, "Teach your children well..."

Sources

Adams, Kelly, Karen C. Lindell, Martin Kohlmeier, and Steven H. Zeisel. "Status of nutrition education in medical schools." The American Journal of Clinical Nutrition 83 (2006), 941S. <http://www.ajcn.org>.

"Alcohol related car accident deaths." Wikipedia: The Free Encyclopedia. Wikimedia Foundation. (accessed 25 Sept. 2011) <http://wikianswers.com/Q/How_many_people_die_from_alcohol_rela...>.

Amarelo, Monica. "EPA proposes bold new limits for tackling 'forever chemicals' in drinking water." Environmental Working Group. ewg.org 14 March 2023.

Aoun, Antoine, Farah Darwiche, Sibelle Al Hayek, and Jacqueline Doumit. "The Fluoride Debate: The Pros and Cons of Fluoridation." ncbi.nlm.nih.gov. 30 Sept. 2018.

Archibold, Randal C. "Arizona Enacts Stringent Law on Immigration." New York Times. 23 Apr.2010. <http://www.nytimes.com/2010/04/24/us/politics/24immig.html?scp=1...>.

Barrows, PhD Julie N., Arthur L. Lipman, PhD, and Catherine J. Bailey, M.Ed., Series Editor: Sebastian Cianci. "Color Additives History." fda.gov (reprinted from Food Safety Magazine Oct./Nov. 2003).

"beta-Carotene." Wikipedia: The Free Encyclopedia. Wikimedia Foundation. (accessed 24 Sept. 2011) <http://en.wikipedia.org/wiki/Beta-Carotene>.

Borenstein, Seth. "Fatso Virus Found. Flab vaccine eyed." New York Post. 21 Aug. 2007:3.

"Brown Sugar." Wikipedia: The Free Encyclopedia. Wikimedia Foundation. (accessed 23 Sept. 2011) <http://en.wikipedia.org/wiki/Brown_sugar>.

Campbell, T. Colin, and Thomas M. Campbell II. The China Study. Dallas: BenBella Books, Inc.,2006.

Cardello, Hank, and Doug Garr. Stuffed. New York: Harper Collins, 2009.

"Chewy Granola Bars." Quaker. n.d. <http://www.quakeroats.com/products/oat-snacks/chewy-granola-bars-le...>.

Childs, Dan. "Study Predicts Obesity Apocalypse by 2030. Experts Weigh in on Fate of Rapidly Fattening Populace." Weight Loss Surgery Specialist. 2 Aug. 2008. <http://weightlosssurgeryspecialists.com>.

"Chocolatey Pretzel Special K Cereal Bar/Special K Cereal Bars." Kellogg. n.d. <http://www.specialk.com/cereal-bars/chocolate-pretzel.>.

Collignon, Andy. "Strategies for Accommodating Obese Patients in an Acute Care Setting." Surgistrategies. 30 Oct. 2008. <http://www.surgistrategies.com/articles/2008/10/strategies-for-accommodating-obese-patients-in-an.aspx>.

Dietz, MD, PhD William H. "Innovative Childhood Obesity Practices." Centers for Disease Control and Prevention. 16 Dec. 2009. <http://www.cdc.gov/washington/testimony/2009/t20091216.htm>.

"Drug and Alcohol Teen Statistics." Red Rock Canyon School. n.d. <http://www.redrock canyonschool.com/article/42>.

"Drugs, Herbs and Supplements." medlineplus.gov/druginformation.html.

Finkelstein, Eric A., and Laurie Zuckerman. The Fattening Of America. Hoboken: John Wiley & Sons, Inc., 2008.

First For Women 18 Jan. 2010, and 25 Apr. 2011: 72, 73, 98.

Fox, Maggie. "Obese Americans now outweigh the merely overweight." Reuters. 9 Jan. 2009. <http://www.reuters.com>.

Friedman, Dr. Michael. "Testimony on Protecting the U.S. Consumer from Food Borne Illnesses." Department of Health and Human Services. 10 May 1996. <http://www.hhs.gov/asl/testify/t960510b.html>.

Fulmer, Melinda. "Do food dyes affect kids' behavior?" Los Angeles Times. 13 Oct. 2008. <http://articles.latimes.com/print/2008/oct/13/health/he-foodcolor13>.

Fumento, Michael. "Porcine Puppies." New York Post. 21 Jan. 2007:25.

"Generally recognized as safe." Wikipedia: The Free Encyclopedia. Wikimedia Foundation. (accessed 30 Jan. 2012) <http://en.wikipedia.org/wiki/Generally_recognized_as_safe>.

"Gingered Blueberry Shortcake." Cooking Light. 2011 <http://search.cookinglight.com/ck-results.html? Ntt=gingered+blueberry...>.

Glassner, Barry. The Gospel of Food. New York: Harper Collins, 2008.

Hall, Susan. "CHOCOLATE...THE HEALTHY INDULGENCE!" Health Sept. 2009: 118.

Hastings, Deborah. "Obesity Finds Niche in American Marketing." BREITBART.COM. 17 Apr. 2006. <http://bsbrigade.com/forums/showthread.php?t=32120>.

Health Sept. 2009: 52, 58, 140, 143, 146, 151, 159.

Hellmich, Nancy. "One-third of kids tip scales wrong way." USA TODAY. 5 Apr. 2006. <http://www.usatoday.com/news/health/2006-04-04-obesity_x.htm>.

"Jif Products." Jif. 28 Apr. 2010. <http://www.jif.com/Products>.

"Kashi Food Products." Food Facts. n.d. <http://www.foodfacts.com/NutritionFacts>.

Knott, Michelle. "Sky-high sugar prices threaten US jobs, warn confectioners." Confectionerynews.com. 15 Sept. 2011 <http://www.confectionerynews.com/content/view/print/561032>.

"Kymaro New Body Shaper." UbuyEZ. n.d. <http://www.ubuyez.com/index.php?main_page=product_info&product...>.

Lee, Bruce Y. "Synthetic Dyes: This Is How Much Kids Are Consuming." Forbes.com. 24 Sept. 2019

Lo, Clifford. "Integrating nutrition as a theme throughout the medical school curriculum." The American Journal of Clinical Nutrition 72 (2000), 882S. <http://www.ajcn.org>.

Lodge, Dr. Henry S. "You can stop 'normal' aging." Parade 18 Mar. 2007: 6, 7.

"Multivitamins." Cerner Multum for Drugs.com. 11 Aug. 2023.

Murphy, Pam. "Percentage of Food Inspected by the FDA." eHow. n.d. <http://www.ehow.com/facts_5548011_percentage-food-inspected-fda.html>.

"National School Lunch Program. Healthy, Hunger-Free Kids Act of 2010, Section 204: Local School Wellness Policies 5-Year Technical Assistance and Guidance Plan." USDA. 20 Sept. 2011. <http://www.fns.usda.gov/cnd/lunch/>.

"Natural Colon Cleansing: Is It Necessary?" WebMD. 25 Aug. 2009. <http://www.webmd.com/balance/natural-colon-cleansing-is-it-necessa...>.

Nestle, Marion. Food Politics: How the Food Industry Influences Nutrition and Health. Berkely and Los Angeles: University of California Press, 2002.

Nestle, Marion. What to Eat. New York: North Point Press, 2006.

Newport, Frank. "U.S. Drinking Rate Edges Up Slightly to 25-Year High." Gallup. 30 July 2010. <http://www.gallup.com/poll/141656/drinking-rate-edges-slightly-year-...>.

"Nutrition's dynamic duos." by Harvard Health Publishing/Harvard Medical School for health.harvard.edu. 1 July 2009.

"Obesity and Genetics." <u>Centers for Disease Control and Prevention</u>. 19 Jan. 2010. <<u>http://www.cdc.gov/Features/Obesity/</u>>.

Ochs, Carol. "CORN SYRUP SOLIDS VS. HIGH FRUCTOSE CORN SYRUP." <u>LIVESTRONG</u>. 14 June 2011. <<u>http://www.livestrong.com/article/315136-corn-syrup-solids-vs-high-fr</u>...>.

"Oxalic Acid and Foods." <u>Oxalic Acid Info</u>. 5 Feb. 2010. <<u>http://oxalicacidinfo.com/</u>>.

Paine, Thomas. "Common Sense." <u>ushistory.org</u>. 14 Feb. 1776. <<u>http://www.ushistory.org/paine/commonsense/singlehtml.htm</u>.>.

"Peter Pan Creamy Peanut Butter." <u>Food Facts</u>. 10 Mar. 2011 <<u>http://www.foodfacts.com/Nutrition</u> Facts/Creamy/Peter-Pan-Creamy-...>.

Peters, MD, Brandon. "What Is Vitamin Toxicity?" 22 Nov. 2023. <u>verywellhealth.com</u>

Pollan, Michael. <u>In Defense Of Food</u>. New York: Penguin Group, 2008.

Sammy, Melissa. "Dangerous duos: 5 supplement combos to avoid." 10 June 2020. <u>mdlinx.com</u>

Seldin, Richard. "The great emptiness that feeds obesity." <u>The Star Ledger</u>. 23 Oct. 2006:17.

"75% Reduced Fat Cheddar." <u>Cabot</u>. n.d. <http://cabotcheese.coop/pages/our_products/product.php?catID...>.

<u>Shape</u> Jan. 2010: 155.

Sharples, Tiffany. "Eating a Bit Less Salt Can Be a Big Health Boon." <u>Time</u>. 12 Mar. 2009. <<u>http://www.time.com/time/printout/0,8816,1884864,00.html</u>>.

Sine, Richard. "Vitamins: Separating Fact From Fiction." 20 Feb. 2006. <u>webmd</u>.

Sissons, Claire. "What is the average percentage of water in the human body?" 27 May 2020. <u>medicalnewstoday</u>.

"Smart Balance Natural and Omega-3 Peanut Butter." <u>Food Facts</u>. 8 Apr. 2010. <<u>http://www.foodfacts.com/NutritionFacts</u>>.

"Smart Choices Program." <u>Smart Choices Program</u>. n.d. <<u>http://www.smartchoicesprogram.com</u>>.

Steward, H. Leighton, et al. <u>The New Sugar Busters!</u>. New York: The Ballantine Publishing Group, 2003.

"Study: 86 Percent of Americans Could Be Obese by 2030." <u>CONSUMERAFFAIRS.COM</u>. 29 July 2008. <<u>http://www.consumeraffairs.com/news04/2008/07obesity_study.html</u>>.

"Sugar." <u>Wikipedia: The Free Encyclopedia</u>. Wikimedia Foundation. (accessed 29 Nov. 2011) <<u>http://en.wikipedia.org/wiki/Sugar</u>>.

Sundaram, Dr. Hema. "The Dangers of Tanning Beds: Five Fast Facts." <u>MySkinCareConnection.com</u>. 2 June 2008. <<u>http://www.healthcentral.com/skin-care/c/75934/24339/beds-fast-facts/pf/</u>>.

Tanner, Lindsey. "How to fight the fat gene: Get lots of physical activity. Try it the Amish way—walk, garden, clean." <u>The Star Ledger</u> 9 Sept. 2008: 36.

"Triglyceride." <u>Wikipedia: The Free Encyclopedia</u>. Wikimedia Foundation. (accessed 23 Sept. 2011) <<u>http://en.wikipedia.org/wiki/Triglyceride</u>>.

"2011 National Diabetes Fact Sheet." <u>Centers for Disease Control and Prevention</u>. 23 May 2011. <<u>http://www.cdc.gov/diabetes/pubs/estimates11.htm#1</u>>.

"Vital Signs Report." <u>Centers for Disease Control and Prevention</u>. 1 Feb. 2011. <<u>http://www.cdc.gov/media/releases/2011/p0201_vitalsigns.html</u>>.

Walsh, Bryan. "What's Really Making America's Children Fat? It's Not Just Genetics." <u>Time</u> 23 June 2008: 73, 74.

Wang, Youfa, May A. Beydoun, Lan Liang, Benjamin Caballero and Shiriki K. Kumanyika. "Will All Americans Become Overweight or Obese? Estimating the Progression and Cost of the US Obesity Epidemic." <u>NATURE.com</u>. 24 July 2008 <<u>http://www.nature.com/oby/journal/v16/n10/full/oby2008351a.html</u>>.

Weil, Dr. Andrew. "Avoid Vegetables with Oxalic Acid?" <u>Weil Lifestyle LLC</u>. 28 Jan. 2008. <<u>http://www.drweil.com/drw/u/QAA400344/Avoid-Vegetables-with-Ox...</u>>.

Wieder, Robert S. "Small World ride revamped for bigger passengers." <u>CalorieLab Calorie Counter News</u>. 3Nov. 2007. <<u>http://calorielab.com/news/2007/10/29/small-world-ride-revamped-for-bigger-passengers/</u>>.

Winik, Lyric Wallwork, David Wallechinsky and Daryl Chen. "Making a Profit Off Kids." <u>Parade</u> 28 Oct. 2007: 10.

Winter, Ruth. <u>A CONSUMER'S DICTIONARY OF FOOD ADDITIVES</u>. New York: Three Rivers Press, 1978.

Zamora, Antonio. "Fats, Oils, Fatty Acids, Triglycerides." <u>Scientific Psychic</u>. <<u>http://www.scientificpsychic.com/fitness/fattyacids.html</u>>.

Zeratsky, R.D., L.D. Katherine. "What is vitamin D toxicity? Should I be worried about taking supplements?" Healthy Lifestyle/Nutrition and healthy eating. <u>mayoclinc.org</u>.

www.ingramcontent.com/pod-product-compliance
Lightning Source LLC
Chambersburg PA
CBHW081530120626
46550CB00009B/2669